HEALTHY
TRANSITIONS

HEALTHY
TRANSITIONS

A WOMAN'S GUIDE TO PERIMENOPAUSE, MENOPAUSE & BEYOND

FOREWORD BY
DR. MARIANNE J. LEGATO,
Founder and Director for
The Partership of Gender-Specific
Medicine at Columbia University

NEIL SHULMAN, M.D.
EDMUND S. KIM, M.D., OB/GYN

Mike,
May your new journey
be blessed & may
you find this useful
for your patients!
ESK

Ⓟ Prometheus Books

59 John Glenn Drive
Amherst, New York 14228-2197

Disclaimer: This book is not intended to substitute for the medical advice of a physician. The reader should regularly consult a physician about matters relating to his or her health and particularly regarding any symptoms that may require medical attention.

Published 2004 by Prometheus Books

Inquiries should be addressed to
Prometheus Books
59 John Glenn Drive
Amherst, New York 14228–2197
VOICE: 716–691–0133, ext. 207
FAX: 716–564–2711
WWW.PROMETHEUSBOOKS.COM

08 07 06 05 04   5 4 3 2 1

Library of Congress Cataloging-in-Publication Data

Shulman, Neil.
    Healthy transitions : a woman's guide to perimenopause, menopause, and beyond / by Neil Shulman, and Edmund S. Kim.
        p. cm.
    Includes bibliographical references and index.
    ISBN 1–59102–150–2
    1. Perimenopause—Popular works. 2. Menopause—Popular works. 3. Middle aged women—Health and hygiene. I. Kim, Edmund. II. Title.
RG186.S6658 2003
618.1'75—dc22

                                                                2003023266

Printed in the United States on acid-free paper

This book is dedicated to my wife, best friend, and soulmate, Sun-Yung; my children, Lucas, Jackson, and Leah, who bring joy to my life; and to my parents, Yong and Lily, who helped guide me to where I am today.

Edmund S. Kim, M.D.

I'd like to salute mom and dad, two souls connected eternally. Dad taught me how to live and how to die. Mom taught me how to love.

Neil Shulman, M.D.

CONTENTS

CHAPTER 2. HOT FLASHES, NIGHT SWEATS, AND DRYNESS, OH MY! 33

CHAPTER 3. MY PERIODS HAVE CHANGED. SHOULD I WORRY? 57

CHAPTER 4. WHAT'S WITH MY MOODS?   89

CHAPTER 5. PACKING ON THE POUNDS   107

CHAPTER 6. NOT IN THE MOOD   125

CHAPTER 7. I CAN'T BE PREGNANT . . .   149

CHAPTER 8. SINGLE AGAIN AND AVOIDING SEXUALLY TRANSMITTED DISEASES 181

CHAPTER 9. HORMONES: THE GOOD, THE BAD, AND THE UGLY 205

CHAPTER 10. NATURAL REMEDIES: WHAT THEY DON'T TELL YOU   **231**

CHAPTER 11. LIFE AFTER MENOPAUSE   **257**

CHAPTER 12. SCREENING TESTS   **283**

FOREWORD

MARIANNE J. LEGATO, M.D.

*M*enopause is a subject fraught with confusion, anxiety, and conflicting opinions about its management. Dr. Shulman and Dr. Kim bring their expertise in making medical information clear and accessible to the layperson—to women in or about to enter menopause. They elucidate the facts women need to understand the symptoms they are experiencing and to decide whether or not to use hormone therapy (HT).

Until 1994 we believed that estrogen treatment was beneficial for all women who could tolerate it as long as there were no absolute contraindications (like breast cancer, for example) to taking it. All that we had learned by watching what happened to women who used hormone therapy convinced us that estrogen not only made the troublesome symptoms of menopause better and prevented bone loss, but cut the risk for coronary artery disease (CAD) in half. It was only in the mid-1990s, when researchers completed the first *prospective, randomized* studies in women, that doubts began to surface. The *prospective, randomized* study is different from the *observational* study: in the former, we assemble a group of volunteers, and randomly assign half of them to the use of the drug being studied, using the other group as "controls" or non-users. Then, after a pre-determined period of time, we compare what happens to users and non-users. Amazingly, the prospective studies on HT indicated that in a small percentage of women above the age of sixty, treatment was associated with a significantly higher incidence of heart attacks, stroke, and blood clots, and in others, breast cancer. On the other hand, fractures and colon cancer were significantly less in women who used estrogen. The new work created an enormous stir and confused many physicians as well as the patients in their care. In fact, the new studies didn't really tell us anything that should have surprised us: we always knew that for a small subset of women, estrogen dangerously increased the tendency of the blood to clot and that such women couldn't tolerate hormone therapy. We also knew that hormone therapy was a hazard for breast cancer in another small subset of women. In our *observational* study, we never captured those vulnerable women. Those who tried and stopped the drug because of side effects were never included in the cohort that was able to begin and continue hormone therapy —the "users." Second, the investigators in the new *prospective* studies chose to give hormone therapy to women well over sixty years of age: we generally begin hormone therapy in women over a decade younger, at the time of menopause. Even the fact that hormone therapy didn't seem to modify or mitigate the progression of coronary artery disease in the older women who made up the group in the prospective studies was not particularly surprising; the arteries of women already affected by coronary artery disease don't have receptors for estrogen any longer, and so can't benefit from hormone therapy. What's more, in mature, well-established coronary artery disease estrogen may actually make plaque (the obstructing lesion that compromises blood flow in the artery affected with atherosclerosis) less stable and likely to rupture.

So at least one decision we now feel comfortable in making that comes out of the newer studies is that hormone therapy shouldn't be started in women with *established coronary* artery disease. As for estrogen's use in younger women for the amelioration of troublesome symptoms of menopause like hot flashes and disturbed sleep patterns, we still think that if there are no absolute contraindications to hormone therapy's use, it can be beneficial if used for as short a period of time as possible and in the lowest doses that will produce improvement in symptoms. We still believe that estrogen is the most effective way to prevent the five- to six-year period of rapid bone loss that follows menopause.

Doctors have always maintained that choosing any treatment is up to not only the patient or not only the doctor: it's a joint decision. The physician's role is to give the patient accurate, complete, and up-to-date information about the proposed intervention and to help her decide whether or not she's going to find it both *safe* and *useful*. This book is a wonderful adjunct to take along to your doctor's office. It's full of information that will help you understand not only what menopause is but your options for the treatment of any symptoms that might be plaguing you.

Marianne J. Legato, M.D., F.A.C.P.
Professor of Clinical Medicine
Columbia University College of Physicians & Surgeons

PREFACE

ANDREA KLEMES, D.O.

My best friend, who is forty-five, became concerned about some weight she had gained. She had a very busy job and ate out frequently. I chalked it up to that and less exercise (no time). Her depression and irritability started to worsen. We talked about adjusting her Prozac dose. When she told me she had not had a period since a minor surgical procedure several months before, I still did not think about the possibility of menopause. I knew that her mother had not gone through menopause until she was fifty-six, so I thought she had plenty of time. I talked to her doctor and suggested that her hormone levels be tested, even though I thought they would be normal and that these issues were just part of her life. Was I ever surprised when her hormone levels showed she had gone through menopause.

I have been taking care of women going through menopause for over tens years. I pride myself in listening and helping those who others ignore. I also think I am pretty good at diagnosing menopause and other hormonal changes. So I was very surprised when my best friend went through menopause right under my nose. It just shows you how hard it is to diagnose even when you are the expert.

Why can a normal life change such as this be so easily missed? Because menopause is not an exact time. Because it is not the same for every woman. Because it is hard to diagnose. Because the symptoms are vague and may manifest in multiple diseases that can occur at this time of life. Because there is no definitive lab test. Because you have to be informed and feel comfortable talking to your doctor.

When I was a medical resident I was taking care of a fifty-two-year-old woman in the intensive care unit who developed vaginal bleeding. My male colleagues were ready to call in a gynecologist to help determine the cause of the bleeding. I asked if she was still having periods. They all said she is over fifty so she must be menopausal. My reply was, "Do not presume!" I found her husband who confirmed that she had not gone through menopause and it was just that time of the month.

Drs. Shulman and Kim have put together an amazing compilation of information that every woman needs to know. They give down-to-earth advice and information in plain language so you can talk to your doctor about your health and know what to ask and what to worry about, or perhaps more importantly what not to worry about. It empowers you to take control of your life.

Why is there a need for this kind of reliable information in this day and age? Years ago women did not talk about menopausal symptoms, partly because they did not live long enough to go through menopause, but partly because these things just weren't discussed with others. Menopause is no longer taboo, but some things still are. There *is* a reason now to talk about female sexual dysfunction, sexually transmitted diseases, and birth control in the older woman. There are more and more perimenopausal single women. Reliable information is needed for all women.

Did you know the average woman now lives over one-third of her life after menopause? It is important to do all you can to maximize your quality of life during this time. Learning what you can do and getting the right information is important for you to be able to do this with your doctor.

Finally, there is a lot of medical research occuring in the area of menopausal health. Large studies on menopausal women have been published recently. As welcome as this new information is, sometimes the results are confusing and even contradictory. Hopefully as these issues are studied further, a better understanding of the treatment options will occur. Research may also provide new and better therapies to treat osteoporosis, female sexual dysfunction, menopausal symptoms, and heart disease. Studies on better ways to control your weight are also being done, which may help with this growing problem.

Ah yes, your weight. This is one of the biggest problems at this time of life and one of the things I get the most complaints about (well, this and hot flashes!). The best thing you can do is to be realistic. Make slow changes that you can maintain. I have patients asking about no-carbohydrate diets. I ask if they can live the rest of their life without carbohydrates. If not, they will gain the weight back when they put the carbohydrates back in their diet. In other words, long-term lifestyle changes are much more important than drastic changes that will help you lose weight in the short term, but not keep it off in the long term.

There is one more very important chapter that I think everyone needs to know about and that is the natural remedy chapter. There are a lot of advertisements about "natural" products and a lot of promises from the companies that make them. Some of these products are not effective and others aren't even safe. It is important to be knowledgeable about them as well any possible interactions with other medications if you are considering using these products.

Information is empowering. It is unsettling to have changes occurring daily in your body, especially if you aren't sure why they are happening. It is also difficult to make decisions about your own health care when you do not have the proper information to draw on. *Healthy Transitions* will help you to know you are not alone, different, or going crazy, which is what many women think when they come to see me. They are very happy when they find out it is *just* menopause! This book will give you the information to compare your experience with that of other women going through menopause and will help you formulate questions for your doctor so that you may pass through this time of transition in a healthy and positive way.

Good luck and enjoy!

Andrea Klemes, D.O.
Fellow of the American College of Endocrinology
Private practice in endocrinology, Tallahassee, Florida
and Senior Regional Medical Director,
Procter & Gamble Pharmaceuticals

ACKNOWLEDGMENTS

*M*any thanks go out to our family, friends, and colleagues who enthusiastically supported us through the creation of this book. Special thanks go to Drs. Lance Wiist and Wilma Lee for their invaluable input and medical expertise in reviewing the book. And special thanks also to Dr. Vincent Ho, my writing partner since medical school on many projects, including children's stories and screenplays, who has challenged and encouraged me to continue to write. Special thanks also to Sun-Yung Kim, my wife, who did the tedious job of tallying the results from the survey and has been an unfailing supporter during this project. Thanks to Linda Regan our editor who helped guide us through this undertaking. Mark Kirby and the people at CYKE, Inc., thank you for your patience and willingness to produce graphics to fit the book and creating the cover. We thank Jason Lunsford for putting the survey online to make it more accessible to health care providers. Thank you Chris Kramer, the production manager, who helped take our words and turn them into this book. Debbie Cimosz, we thank you for helping pull together the tables in this book. And finally, to all those women who are experiencing or have experienced perimenopause and menopause who provided the quotes we have sprinkled throughout the book, many thanks. The book could not have been what it is without the effort and dedication of all involved. We thank you all.

INTRODUCTION

*M*enopause, like puberty, is a rite of passage for women. And like puberty, it happens only once so that you can't know for certain what to anticipate. So for years, women have turned to family, friends, and health care professionals to give them advice as they feel the stirrings of the transition to menopause—a stage called perimenopause. The main problem with turning to family and friends for advice is that their information is often ambiguous, contradictory, and at times wrong. Where can you go for reliable information?

Physicians are educators. We teach individuals on a one-to-one basis what is happening with their bodies and minds and the ways to maintain their health. However, as physicians, the number of people we can educate is limited to those we can actually see. And because of a number of factors, such as time constraints and embarrassment, a woman may not ask all the questions she has or she may not have them completely answered. This book has grown out of our desire to reach out and to provide the facts to more women than we could through our practices.

We will address a range of issues and concerns that we have seen women face as they go through the transition to menopause and beyond. Our goal is to effectively communicate the answers to questions you may have and provide strategies to help ease you through this phase of life. This can be a period of growth, knowledge, and empowerment. You may not have control over all the symptoms and issues you face, but how you deal with them is completely under your control. It is our aim not only to help you stay in control of this phase, but to empower you to enjoy your life—both physically and emotionally—to the fullest.

Sprinkled throughout the book are quotes from women who are experiencing or have experienced perimenopause and menopause. Their words will give you a glimpse into the personal feelings and individual experiences that women have during this time of transition. Read and enjoy.

CHAPTER 1

PERIMENOPAUSE TO MENOPAUSE
The Transition

*M*enopause. It means so many things to so many people. Why does this word elicit such a wide range of responses? Menopause is not a disease. It is not a medical condition that needs to be treated. It is a natural stage of a woman's life, like puberty. And puberty is not a disease (though some may think it is). Like puberty, menopause is a stage of life that all women will pass through. And like puberty, each woman is affected in a unique way by this change.

Some women welcome an end to their monthly periods. Others are disturbed by the changes they are experiencing as they go through this transition. Still others are worried by fears that this is the first stage of deteriorating health and a loss of their youth. Psychological and social factors also enter into the picture at this time, such as changes in relationships, financial concerns, and other stressors that have an impact on how each woman perceives this transition.

As practicing physicians in gynecology and internal medicine, we have had the privilege of being invited into the lives and minds of thousands of women. As we have gotten to know and follow them through their lives, a number of recurrent issues keep popping up, especially in those women in their late thirties until they reach menopause. During this time, women notice a number of changes in their bodies and their minds. This transition before menopause is called perimenopause.

PERIMENOPAUSE AND PUBERTY

It helps to think of perimenopause as reverse puberty. During puberty, there is an increase in the sex hormones that leads to changes in a woman's mind, body, and emotions. It can be a confusing time adjusting to the changes these hormones cause. After puberty, the female sex hormones generally fall into a routine monthly cycle except during pregnancy. Then in the late thirties or early forties these hormones start to go through another change. This time, instead of the hormones rising as they do during puberty, they fall until they drop to a new lower level as a woman goes through menopause.

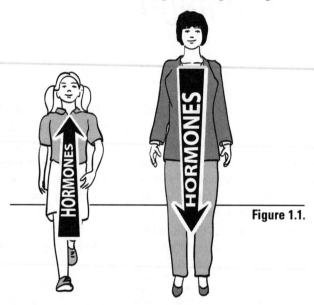

Figure 1.1.

MENOPAUSE AND AGING

Many people associate menopause with aging. Why is this? About a hundred years ago the life expectancy for a woman was about fifty. The average age of menopause was and still is around fifty-one. So at that time, many women died before they completely went through menopause. In the early 1900s, menopause was potentially a signal that a woman's life was close to the end.

Fast forward a century. Now women live into their eighties and beyond. A woman born today can expect to live over a third of her life after she goes through menopause. So instead of marking the end, menopause

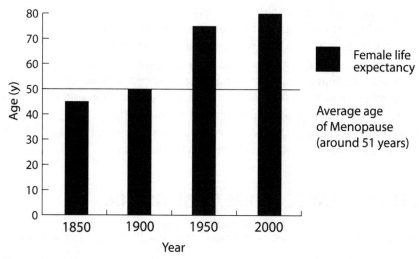

Figure 1.2. *Life expectancy for a woman in relation to average age of menopause.*

now marks only the beginning of another phase of her life. And in this stage of life, many women feel more confident and empowered. By this time, many women have become comfortable with who they are and what they have accomplished and are looking forward to their futures. Other women, however, are still struggling with losses and other major negative life changes that can have an impact on their physical and mental health.

MENOPAUSE AND HEALTH

In the past, and even now, many physical and mental problems were erroneously blamed on the hormonal changes associated with menopause. The medical community unfortunately perpetuated these stereotypes that have pervaded our social and cultural beliefs. A. M. Farnham published a paper in 1887 called "Uterine disease as a factor in the production of insanity" and wrote:

> The ovaries, after long years of service, have not the ability of retiring in graceful old age, but become irritated, transmit their irritation to the abdominal ganglia, which in turn transmit the irritation to the brain, producing disturbances in the cerebral tissue exhibiting themselves in extreme nervousness or in an outburst of actual insanity.[1]

Why does the false association between menopause and such problems persist? Perhaps at this stage of life, many women go through major external changes in their lives. Many of these changes, especially in the past, were negative changes: illness and death in their spouse, friends, or relatives; their own declining health (remember, the average woman in 1900 only lived to fifty); loss of financial security; loss of children as they moved away; need to care for aging parents; and the realization that many dreams would not be fulfilled. The stress of these negative events accounted for many of the problems blamed entirely on hormones.

PERIMENOPAUSE: A TIME OF TRANSITION

Strong cultural and social issues may still exist that can influence how a woman perceives this transition through menopause. In our current cultural climate that worships youth and sexual attractiveness, there is a certain fear of aging. In other cultures, the types of symptoms and problems differ. For example, while up to 85 percent of Caucasian women experience hot flashes, less than 25 percent of Japanese or Chinese women experience them.[2] This highlights the fact that there are a number of factors involved in the way women feel during this transition.

Perimenopause is therefore not only a physical transition brought about by decreasing hormone levels, but also a psychological and social time of change. And it is this combination of physical, mental, emotional, and spiritual changes that for many women trigger a feeling of unease, of being unsettled. A woman's individual traits, her cultural background, her strengths and weaknesses, and the individual challenges she faces at this time help determine how she will view this period of her life.

FACTORS THAT INFLUENCE AGE OF MENOPAUSE

Menopause may also be induced and thus occur earlier than expected. The surgical removal of both ovaries or damage to the ovaries from radiation or chemotherapy can make the ovaries fail earlier. When menopause is caused by the surgical removal of the ovaries, it is called *surgical menopause*.

Other factors may affect when a woman goes through menopause. Women who smoke go through menopause about one and a half years earlier than women who don't smoke. Smoking more and for a longer time tends to make menopause occur earlier. Even women who have quit smoking may still go through menopause earlier.[3]

There also seems to be a genetic component to early menopause. Women whose mothers went through early menopause are more likely to go through early menopause themselves. Other factors associated with earlier menopause include low body weight, never having children, vegetarian diet, living at high altitudes, malnourishment, toxic chemical exposure, and treatment of childhood cancer with radiation or chemotherapy.[4]

Later menopause is associated with having had more pregnancies and being overweight.[5]

SOME DEFINITIONS

The language concerning menopause can be confusing since many times you will hear words in the press or in books used inappropriately. Here are the meanings of some commonly used terms in reference to menopause.

Menopause is defined as the time when a woman stops menstruating because of a loss of the functioning of her ovaries. "Natural" menopause is recognized only after there is no more menstrual bleeding for one year. The average age of menopause in this country is fifty-one, with most women going through menopause between the ages of forty-eight to fifty-five.[6] It has been estimated that in the United States, close to five thousand women enter menopause every day. Because of the baby-boomer generation, more women than ever are experiencing menopause.

Perimenopause is the time leading up to menopause when women start to have symptoms related to this time of transition. This is the word that would describe the time when many women say that they are "going through menopause." The average age at which women start the perimenopausal period is 47.5 years. Perimenopause usually lasts two to seven years in most women. It begins when a woman starts to have symptoms related to menopause and continues until a year after her last period.

Premenopause is a confusing term because it has been used in a number of ways. Some people use it synonymously with perimenopause to describe the time before menopause, though this word is also used by some to connote the entire reproductive time period before menopause. Because of the lack of a standard definition of this word, if it is used, you should find out exactly what it means in a given situation.

Premature menopause refers to women going through menopause early. Some people define premature menopause as experiencing menopause before age thirty-five while others use age forty as a marker. About 1 percent of women go through menopause under the age of forty.[7] This is due to the ovaries in these women failing prematurely. This may be caused by genetic factors, autoimmune problems, or other medical reasons.

Postmenopause is the time after the last menstrual period and lasts for the rest of a woman's life. It differs from the definition of menopause in that menopause is a single point in time whereas postmenopause refers to the span of time covering a woman's life after menopause.

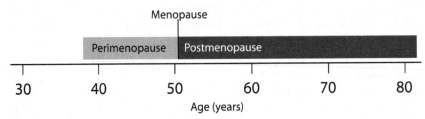

Figure 1.3.

HEALTH CARE PROVIDERS

Women may be seen by a physician, whether it is a gynecologist, family physician, or internist, or perhaps a nurse practitioner, physician assistant, or certified nurse-midwife for their health care needs. A gynecologist is a medical doctor who has completed four years of training specializing in women's health after medical school. After graduating from medical school, an internist has completed three years of training in adult medicine, whereas a family physician has completed three years of training in treating people of all ages, from newborn to old age.

A nurse practitioner is a registered nurse who has usually completed a program where he or she receives additional training in treating patients that grants either a certificate or a master's degree. A physician assistant is a health care professional licensed to practice medicine with physician supervision. He or she has completed a program that runs an average of twenty-six months. A certified nurse-midwife is a health care provider who has been trained in both nursing and midwifery at an accredited program and has passed a national certifying exam. Nurse practitioners, physician assistants, and certified nurse-midwives generally work under the supervision of a physician.

For the rest of this chapter and in other parts of this book, when we refer to a physician, it may mean any of these health care providers whom you may see for your medical care. However, not all health care providers may do all of the tests we discuss in this book. Which tests they do depend on their training. Because of this, it is important to know what their training is. Whoever you see, you should bring up any questions or concerns you have.

What should you be doing during this time? What can be expected? What are your options? In the following chapters we will explore the mystery of this transition as you pass through the threshold to another fascinating phase of your life. You will learn what is normal and what is not, to separate fact from fiction, and discover ways that you can make this a time of growth, knowledge, and empowerment so that you emerge through this period healthier, happier, and stronger.

CHAPTER 2

HOT FLASHES, NIGHT SWEATS, AND DRYNESS, OH MY!

*M*any women are so concerned about menopause that they overlook the changes that occur *before* menopause in the perimenopausal period. Part of the reason for this has been that this period, until recently, has not been widely recognized or discussed. Symptoms during perimenopause were often misinterpreted and blamed on the patient or her life circumstances.

We are now beginning to understand that changes start earlier than previously thought. Traditionally, perimenopause has been defined as the beginning of hormonal changes that manifest themselves as symptoms such as irregular bleeding. We are now starting to see that changes in the ovaries start as early as the midthirties. This may explain why more subtle alterations relating to changing hormone levels are experienced before the typical hot flashes or irregular periods occur. For example, worsening PMS and lessening of libido may be related to these earlier hormonal changes.

IS THERE A TEST TO SEE IF YOU ARE IN THE PERIMENOPAUSAL PERIOD?

Unfortunately there is currently no test to tell if a woman is in the perimenopausal period or close to menopause. Many people think that since hormone levels are changing, that a blood test can be done to see if there is a drop in hormone levels. However, hormone levels such as estrogen vary from day to day and the normal range is quite broad. Typically during the perimenopausal period, the estrogen levels stay within the normal range, even when a woman has significant symptoms.

FSH (Follicle Stimulating Hormone) is produced by the pituitary gland, a small gland at the base of the brain. It stimulates the ovaries to produce estrogen. When estrogen levels are low, FSH goes up to stimulate the ovaries to produce more estrogen. When women go through menopause and their estrogen levels fall, FSH rises to high levels trying to stimulate the ovaries to produce estrogen. However, the ovaries at this time cannot respond to the FSH so estrogen levels stay low and the FSH stays high.

However, since there can be a variation in hormone levels, there have been times when a woman's estrogen and FSH levels seemed to show that a woman had gone through menopause only to have her periods start again. When these hormones were checked again, they were back to the normal range. So a single blood test may not be a completely reliable indicator that a woman has completely gone through menopause.

> *I wish they wouldn't look at age but just listen to symptoms because everyone is different. I started having my first symptoms at age thirty-nine and they told me I was too young. By the time I was forty-two, I was done.*
>
> *—Sharon Anderson*

SYMPTOMS OF PERIMENOPAUSE

What are some of the symptoms experienced during perimenopause?

- Changes in menstrual cycles
- Hot flashes and night sweats
- Sleep problems
- Vaginal changes
- Bladder problems
- Breast changes
- Headaches

- Memory and cognitive changes
- Fatigue
- Sexual changes
- Depression
- Moodiness

The symptoms any given woman has are very individualized and may come and go from perimenopause through menopause and beyond. Some women experience a few minor symptoms, while others suffer severe symptoms. Some symptoms worsen then diminish with time, while others may gradually grow more troublesome.

> *As of forty years of age my periods have ceased—it's wonderful—have never had hot flashes or any of the horrors of menopause most ladies experience. Life is great.*
>
> *—Deborah Wallace*

HOT FLASHES AND NIGHT SWEATS

We know a perimenopausal nurse who called her hot flashes "power surges." Hot flashes are a sudden feeling of warmth or heat resulting from an increase in blood flow to the skin. Hot flashes are especially intense on the upper body and face, causing flushing of the skin. The skin actually does get warmer and the loss of heat through the skin and the sweating caused by the hot flash leads to cooling which can cause chills. When this happens at night, it is often referred to as night sweats. They usually last from a few seconds to several minutes and may happen only once or up to several times a night.

> *I'm HOT and need sleep. I could heat my entire house. My kids complain, the windows are frosted (no lie!), and my son keeps a floor heater in his bedroom. My thermostat is at sixty degrees or below (even in the winter). The neighbor once asked my husband why the air conditioner runs in the winter.*
>
> *—Vangie Davis*

How Common Are Hot Flashes?

Hot flashes are the second most common perimenopausal symptom after irregular periods experienced by up to 85 percent of women in this country.[1] Some women have no hot flashes, others experience them infrequently, but for 15 percent, they can be very frequent and debilitating, occurring throughout the day. Hot flashes usually continue for three to five years, but as many as 25 to 50 percent of women may have them for longer than five years.[2]

Hot flashes differ among cultures. Women in other cultures including Mayan and Asian-Indian report relatively few hot flashes.[3] The reason for this disparity could be related to biological, nutritional, lifestyle, psychological, and social factors. Regardless of the reasons, hot flashes are a symptom experienced by most women in the United States and can have a significant impact on their lives.

Hot flashes or night sweats can cause sleep problems. Night sweats, by awakening a woman throughout the night, can disturb her sleep patterns, leading to fatigue and sleepiness during the day. This can, in turn, produce decreased energy, irritability, loss of concentration and focus, and depressive symptoms. Hot flashes themselves can interfere with daily activities. They are also associated with palpitations and feelings of anxiety.

Potential Triggers for Hot Flashes

- A warm environment
- Stress
- Hot or spicy foods
- Hot drinks
- Alcohol
- Caffeine
- Certain medications

What triggers hot flashes is not completely understood. Whether or not it is truly caused by low or fluctuating hormone levels is unclear. As uncomfortable as hot flashes can be, fortunately, they are not a danger to your health. However, because they can significantly affect the quality of life for some women, different treatment options are available.

What Can I Do about Hot Flashes?

The simplest strategy is to dress in layers so that you can add or remove layers to stay comfortable and to keep yourself cooler by using a fan or setting the thermostat lower. Avoiding the above triggers is another way to minimize hot flashes.

> *I never wore a silk nightgown until I was forty-six years old and experiencing night sweats. Now I own silk blouses and silk scarves. Not only is it a luxurious fabric, it's cool.*
> *—Virginia Sharp Franz*

Exercise

Exercise may help decrease hot flashes. Women who exercised three or more times a week experienced fewer hot flashes, had less negative moods, a smaller decrease in sexual desire, and less problems with memory and concentration.[4] Not to mention that it's good for your heart and bones and who knows what else. If there is one thing you can do for yourself that will do the most for your overall health, it's regular exercise. This doesn't mean you have to join a gym and sign up for classes. It's as simple as putting on a pair of comfortable shoes and walking out your front door. (Check out chapter 13 for more on the benefits of exercise.)

> *I began to exercise more earnestly to lose weight—but as my exercise increased, my hot flashes vanished. Now regardless of tasks needing to be done, rain or shine, exercise comes first!*
> *—Kim Baraona*

Stop Smoking

Women who smoke have more severe and frequent hot flashes than non-smokers. There is a trend toward more hot flashes in women who smoked more cigarettes over a longer period of time. Former smokers had a modest increase in hot flashes over nonsmokers but not as severe as current smokers.[5]

Weight

Heavier women have more frequent and severe hot flashes during perimenopause. However, after menopause, heavier women tend to have fewer hot flashes.[6] So weight loss may help reduce hot flashes during perimenopause but may make them worse after menopause. Weight control is still beneficial for other health reasons (see chapter 5).

Deep Breathing, Relaxation Techniques, and Other Natural Remedies

Deep breathing and other relaxation techniques may also be helpful with hot flashes. Because of their other potential benefits, such as reducing stress and anxiety, relaxation methods are useful to learn. These options as well as other natural remedies are discussed in detail in chapter 10.

Estrogen

Estrogen, a hormone, has been the mainstay of treatment, but recent studies have made women more wary of using it. Estrogen is very effective in helping reduce hot flashes. Estrogen also has some other beneficial effects such as decreasing vaginal dryness, strengthening bones, and reducing the risk of colon cancer. But estrogen may increase the risk of certain problems including blood clots in the legs, heart attacks, and stroke. Progestins (synthetic compounds that act like progesterone) have been used alone and have been found to be helpful with hot flashes. But progestins can also cause problems. (See chapter 9 to learn more about hormones.)

Antidepressants

Serotonin reuptake inhibitors (SSRIs) are a class of antidepressants that include fluoxetine (Prozac), paroxetine (Paxil), sertraline (Zoloft), venlafaxine (Effexor), citalopram (Celexa), and others. Recent studies have shown that fluoxetine (Prozac), paroxetine (Paxil), and venlafaxine (Effexor) can reduce hot flashes.[7] However, these medications have side effects including insomnia, nausea, fatigue, dizziness, suppression of libido, and increased difficulty having orgasm.[8]

Clonidine

Clonidine, a medication used mostly for high blood pressure, has been shown to modestly reduce hot flashes in some studies when compared to placebo, but other studies have not shown this benefit.[9] It is available as a pill or a patch. The main side effects of clonidine are dry mouth, constipation, and drowsiness. It may decrease blood pressure so that you may feel very light-headed and dizzy when you stand.[10]

Bellergal

Bellergal, a combination of belladonna, ergotamine, and Phenobarbital, has been used to reduce hot flashes. However, the effectiveness of this treatment seems to last less than eight weeks. In one study, Bellergal Retard was found to reduce hot flashes greater than placebo after two and four weeks of treatment. After eight weeks, it was no longer more effective than placebo.[11]

> *I'm forty-four and have been "hot" for a few years. . . . He [my physician] proceeded to tell me that I had two choices—I could come to see him and get on medication or I could move to Alaska. I am now on medication, but I'm still thinking how much I'd like fresh salmon.*
>
> *—Kathy R. Cox*

Medical Problems That Can Cause Hot Flashes

Certain medical problems such as hyperthyroidism can cause hot flashes at any age. Hyperthyroidism is a medical condition where your thyroid gland produces too much thyroid hormone. You can have symptoms such as:

- Heat intolerance
- Sweating
- Palpitations
- Diarrhea
- Tremors
- Nervousness or anxiety
- Weight loss

Sometimes these symptoms may be attributed to perimenopause or menopause and this medical condition could be missed. If there is any question that hyperthyroidism is causing your symptoms, a blood test can be done to detect this problem.

SLEEP PROBLEMS

A survey by the National Sleep Foundation showed that perimenopausal and postmenopausal women slept less, reported more symptoms of insomnia, and were twice as likely to use prescription sleep medications than women who had not started perimenopause.[12] Sleep problems, either due to a lack of sleep or poor quality of sleep, can cause fatigue, irritability, and decrease motivation, and can also affect memory and the ability to concentrate and perform work or other tasks.

You can have problems falling asleep and/or waking in the middle of the night and having problems falling back to sleep. The most common complaint among menopausal women is frequent awakenings during the night.[13]

Causes of Sleep Problems

The problems with sleep could be related to night sweats or life stressors (many women have more stress at this time of their lives) or medical sleep disorders such as sleep apnea (a condition when a person stops breathing repeatedly through the night, usually caused by a temporary blockage of the airway). All of the above become more common after menopause. However, it is unclear if these problems such as sleep apnea are directly related to hormones.

Nonetheless, night sweats, which researchers know are related to hormones, are the most obvious link between hormones and sleep disturbances. The night sweats can be so severe that some women have to change their wet bedclothes and sheets. Hot flashes and night sweats also diminish the quality of sleep, even if you don't wake up.[14]

Here are some things you can do to help with nighttime hot flashes:

- Keep your home and bedroom cool, especially when preparing for bed
- Use an electric fan even in winter
- Do not take warm baths near bedtime

- Wear cotton or silk nightclothes; use cotton sheets
- Keep a thermos of ice water to drink at bedside
- If sharing an electric blanket, use one with dual controls
- Keep a log of hot flashes for two weeks and note what triggers hot flashes
- Learn to breathe from the abdomen, not the chest. Slow breathing can help with hot flashes

Poor Quality of Sleep

Menopausal women without hot flashes also complain of sleep problems. Sometimes women will complain of the fatigue, irritability, moodiness, and other consequences of the sleep disruption instead of focusing on their poor quality of sleep. If fatigue is the main complaint, your thyroid and iron levels should be checked to ensure that the fatigue is not caused by a hypothyroid conditions (low thyroid level) or anemia (low blood count).

*Hyper*thyroid (too much thyroid hormone) conditions can cause heat intolerance and sweating, which may mimic menopausal symptoms, but there is usually no fatigue, whereas *hypo*thyroid (not enough thyroid hormone) conditions generally cause fatigue, which can also be seen during perimenopause but not because of any sleep problems. Thyroid problems do become more common as you get older. But because it is difficult at times to determine whether the fatigue felt during the day is related to sleep problems or some other medical condition such as hypothyroidism, blood tests should be done to rule out these medical problems.

Medications Can Cause Insomnia

Certain medications can also promote insomnia, including:[15]

- Clonidine (blood pressure medicine)
- Propranolol (blood pressure medicine)
- Atenolol (blood pressure medicine)
- Pindolol (blood pressure medicine)
- Atrovent (used for asthma and allergies)
- Ritalin (used for attention deficit disorder)
- Albuterol (asthma medicine)
- Theophylline (asthma medicine)
- Pseudoephedrine (found in over-the-counter cold and sinus medicines)

- Phenylpropanolamine (found in over-the-counter cold and sinus medicines)
- Medroxyprogesterone (a progesterone type compound)
- Phenytoin (antiseizure medicine)
- Nicotine
- Caffeine

If you have started taking a new medication, even something over the counter, and you notice problems with sleep, check with your physician to see if this could be the cause of your sleeping problems.

GOOD SLEEP HABITS

- *Keep regular hours for meals and sleep*
- *Nap less than thirty minutes a day*
- *Exercise regularly*
- *Go outdoors for thirty minutes or more each day, especially in late afternoon*
- *Limit caffeine and alcohol*
- *Restrict liquids near bedtime*

What Can You Do about Sleep Problems?

Go Outside

Going outdoors and getting exposed to daylight is the best way to regulate your circadian rhythm. The circadian rhythm is your body's natural internal clock that aligns your body's activity level to the time of day. For example, during the night, your blood pressure, heart rate, and temperature all drop when you are sleeping. Even if you are awake at that time of night, those vital functions still drop. The daylight exposure helps reset your internal clock.

People who aren't exposed to natural light, especially those in an institutional setting, may disrupt their sleep-wake cycles because their internal clock is not reset on a regular basis. Going outside is good for other reasons such as helping you produce vitamin D, which helps you absorb calcium (good for your bones). Some people who aren't exposed to enough daylight have problems with depression. This is called seasonal affective disorder (SAD) and is seen more commonly in the northern part of the country during the winter when there is much less daylight. When you do go outside, especially during the summer, you should protect your skin from the damaging effects of the sun.

Exercise

Exercising for thirty to forty minutes four times a week has been shown to help shorten the time to fall asleep, to increase the amount of time sleeping, and to improve sleep quality. However, you should avoid exercising near bedtime because it can take a while for your body's metabolism to slow down afterward, which may make it more difficult to fall asleep.

Sleeping Pills

Sleeping medications should be avoided as long-term solutions to sleep problems. The most commonly used class of medications are called benzodiazepines. They do help you fall asleep, but they can increase the likelihood of daytime drowsiness, confusion, and falls, which may lead to injury.

The problem with long-term use is that this class of medications is addictive and your body can become dependent on these medications to help you sleep. If you use them for long periods of time, you can also build up a tolerance so that you need to take more and more of the medication to help you sleep. If you stop taking these sleeping pills after being on them for a long period of time, you could go through withdrawal and have severe sleeping problems until your body readjusts to life without these medications.

Estrogen

Estrogen has been shown to be helpful in reducing the time to fall asleep, the number of nighttime awakenings, and increase the amount of time spent in deep sleep.[16] As noted, estrogen has been shown to be very effective in reducing hot flashes and night sweats and this is one way estrogen may help improve sleep. Estrogen has other benefits but also risks (which are further discussed in chapter 9).

Antidepressants

Certain antidepressants such as doxepin (Sinequan), trimipramine, and amitriptyline (Elavil) are sedating and have been prescribed to help with sleep. Serotonin reuptake inhibitors (SSRIs) do not cause sedation but may help with insomnia related to depression. They have also been used to help with sleep problems. However, the effectiveness of antidepressants in treating sleep problems, not related to a mood disorder such as depression, is unclear and sometimes these medications themselves can cause insomnia.[17]

Melatonin

Melatonin is a hormone produced by the pineal gland and is released only at night. It has been used to help people with jet lag and to improve sleep. Studies in healthy adults over fifty have shown that taking melatonin thirty minutes before bedtime may improve sleep with few apparent side effects.[18] However, the efficacy and safety of long-term melatonin use has not been studied at this time partly because it is considered a dietary supplement. (For more information on dietary supplements, please see chapter 10.)

VAGINAL CHANGES

As you go through menopause, vaginal changes occur. The vagina has one of the highest concentrations of estrogen receptors in the body. Estrogen receptors are what estrogen attaches to on a cell to affect that tissue. Having a higher concentration of estrogen receptors makes that area more sensitive to a drop in estrogen levels. After menopause, with the drop in estrogen levels, the vaginal lining becomes thinner and less elastic. The vagina becomes shorter, narrower, and more easily irritated. It also creates less lubrication, which can have an impact on sexual functioning.

Within five years of menopause, most women will notice some degree of change, though it will not cause problems for all women. You may feel dryness, irritation, or itching in the vagina or the areas outside the opening of the vagina. (For more information about these changes, please see chapter 6.)

Yeast Infections and Bacterial Vaginosis

A less obvious change is the change in the vaginal environment. The pH of the vagina becomes less acidic and can lead to more vaginal infections such as yeast infections and bacterial vaginosis. Bacterial vaginosis is caused by an overgrowth of bacteria that normally grow only in small amounts in the vagina. The main bacteria in the vagina is lactobacilli. It suppresses the growth of yeast and these other bacteria. If the pH changes, the lactobacilli die off and the yeast or other bacteria overgrow, causing discharge, irritation, and/or an odor.

Yeast infections and bacterial vaginosis can have similar symptoms. Your health care provider can look at your discharge under a microscope and usually tell you what is causing the problem. Yeast infections are treated with either antiyeast creams placed in the vagina, or a pill that is taken by mouth. Bacterial vaginosis is treated by an antibiotic cream in the vagina or an antibiotic pill.

Vaginal Irritants

The vaginal area can become more sensitive because of these changes. Certain soaps, bath gels, bubble baths, detergents, or other things that come in contact with this area may now cause irritation, even though they didn't cause irritation in the past. Other skin changes such as lichen sclerosis are more common after menopause and can cause itching and irritation. You will need to be examined and possibly have a biopsy done if you have a problem that persists.

BLADDER PROBLEMS

Urinary incontinence (the involuntary leaking of urine), bladder infections, urinating more frequently, having the urge to urinate even when your bladder isn't full are some of the bladder problems that increase in frequency during perimenopause and menopause. The base of the bladder, the urethra (the opening to your bladder), and the vagina have the highest concentration of estrogen receptors in the body. As the estrogen levels drop, this may affect the bladder in a way that contributes to these problems.

As many as 10 to 30 percent of women between ages fifty and sixty-four are affected by urinary incontinence.[19] Urine can accidentally leak out when coughing, sneezing, laughing, jumping, running, or lifting. This is called stress incontinence which occurs when you put more pressure on the bladder.

Some women have urge incontinence, where they have the urge to urinate and leak as their bladder contracts and tries to push the urine out. Some women leak during intercourse or with orgasm (see chapter 6). Or the urine leakage could be caused by a mixture of these two types of incontinence. Urinary incontinence increases with age, and decreasing estrogen levels may be one of the factors contributing to this problem.

Stress Urinary Incontinence

Stress urinary incontinence is leaking of urine caused when you put stress or push on the bladder. Weakening of the pelvic muscles from natural aging and damage from childbirth can contribute to urinary incontinence. The muscles around the opening of your bladder and vagina form part of the pelvic floor. Like any other muscle, these muscles get weaker with age, especially if you don't exercise them. Childbirth also can stretch and tear these muscles and the nerves that go to these muscles, further weakening them. Kegel's exercises help strengthen the pelvic muscles.

Kegel's Exercises

The last time you probably remember doing Kegel's exercises was during pregnancy. If you don't remember how to do your Kegel's exercises, next time you urinate, try to stop the flow of urine. Those are the muscles you want to strengthen. You will want to tighten just your pelvic muscles for a couple of seconds, not your stomach or butt muscles. If you feel yourself tightening your stomach muscles at the same time, try to breathe out, sing, or talk while you are doing the Kegel's exercise. This will help you tighten the right muscle. Once you figure out how to do these exercises, don't do them while urinating but at other times.

Ideally, you will want to do twenty sets of five a day (a total of one hundred every day). Every time you are at a stop light or see a commercial on television, do a set of five. Don't expect to see improvement right away. It takes about three months of consistent daily Kegel's to see a significant change. Kegel's are just like any other exercise. You don't expect to be stronger a couple of days after starting a workout program at the gym. Kegel's are easy to do, have no downsides, and if you do eventually need surgery, doing Kegel's improves the outcome. So what are you waiting for? Do a set now and keep doing them.

Pessaries

Other options to help with stress urinary incontinence are pessaries and surgery. Pessaries are basically different shaped objects made out of rubber or silicone that are placed in the vagina. They are used to hold up the bladder or uterus if they start to push out of the vagina and they put pressure on the bladder neck to help prevent leaking of urine.

Pessaries can take some manual dexterity to place and to remove. The placement and removal may be uncomfortable, but it should not cause pain or discomfort when it is in place. Pessaries need to be removed periodically to be cleaned. They can cause ulcerations or sores on the vaginal wall, a vaginal discharge which may have an odor, and rarely, if left in place for too long, can erode through the bladder or rectum causing urine or stool to leak through the vagina.

Surgery for Stress Urinary Incontinence

Many different types of surgeries have been tried to help with stress urinary incontinence. They all basically try to support the neck of the bladder so that there is more pressure on the urethra (the tube that empties the bladder) to keep the urine from leaking. Surgery is good for stress incontinence, but can cause long-term irritation of the bladder, making you feel the urge to urinate even when your bladder isn't full. Surgery can also lead to problems with emptying your bladder.

Urge Incontinence

Urge incontinence occurs when the bladder contracts or tightens up and pushes urine out. When your bladder is filled to a certain point, your bladder contracts to push the urine out and that's when you feel the urge to urinate. If your pelvic muscles are strong enough, you can hold the urine in until you get to the bathroom or until the bladder walls relax. When your bladder relaxes, you feel the urge to urinate subside. Surgery is not a good option for urge incontinence because the problem is not with the neck of the bladder.

Certain things like caffeine, alcohol, acidic foods, and carbonated drinks can irritate the bladder, making it want to contract even when your bladder isn't very full. Avoiding those things that irritate your bladder can help with urinary urgency and the need to urinate frequently and can also help with urge incontinence. Strengthening your pelvic muscles with Kegel's exercises is also helpful.

Bladder Training

Bladder training programs have been shown to be effective in treating urge incontinence. What you are trying to do is train your bladder to hold more urine and to keep from leaking when you do have the urge to urinate. Women with urge incontinence have diminished bladder capacity: their bladder doesn't want to hold as much urine as it did in the past. Once their bladder fills to a certain point, even though it's not full, it wants to push the urine out.

One method is to have a certain voiding schedule, where you urinate on a regular basis, for example, every hour. Once you are able to consistently go one hour without leaking, you increase the interval between urinations by five to ten minutes. When you can consistently go this new interval without leaking, you increase the interval again. You keep doing this until you can go for two to three hours without leaking.

The other method is to learn strategies to prevent incontinence. You learn to do Kegel's exercises (tighten your pelvic floor). Once you learn how to contract those muscles which may or may not involve the use of biofeedback, you then change your response when you feel the urge to urinate. Instead of immediately rushing to the bathroom (which most women do to avoid leaking but unfortunately tends to make you leak more), you wait.

Try to sit and relax your body and contract your pelvic floor muscles repeatedly until the bladder relaxes and the urge to urinate subsides. Then get up and go to the bathroom at a normal pace. This behavioral method has been shown to decrease the number of incontinence episodes by up to 80 percent and was more effective than treatment with medication.[20] Interestingly, the use of biofeedback did not improve the outcome.[21]

Medications for Urinary Incontinence

Medications are also useful in helping with urge incontinence. The two most commonly used medications are oxybutynin (Ditropan) and tolterodine (Detrol), which help relax the bladder. The main problems with these medications are dry mouth, which is the most common bothersome side effect. Other side effects include constipation, upset stomach, headache, dizziness, blurry vision, and nausea.[22] Tolterodine generally has fewer of these side effects.

Urinary urgency (the urge to urinate) and urinary frequency (urinating more frequently) can become bothersome even without any leakage of urine. The urge to urinate can occur so frequently that it interferes with sleep and daily activities. Treatment is similar to that for urge incontinence. Bladder training exercises to increase the interval between voids, and Kegel's exercises (pelvic floor exercises) which are done until the urge passes help increase bladder capacity. Physicians may prescribe the above medications if the symptoms become severe.

Urinary Tract Infections

Older women are more likely to get urinary tract infections (UTIs), also known as bladder infections. They are also more likely to have recurrences.

Certain factors increase the risk of urinary tract infections, including:[23]

- Urinary incontinence (leaking of urine)
- Cystocele (having your bladder "drop" or bulge into the vagina)
- Inability to completely empty your bladder (it's easier for bacteria to grow in the bladder if all the urine isn't flushed out when voiding)
- History of bladder surgery
- Lack of estrogen
- Diabetes (which decreases your body's ability to fight infection)

Most of these risk factors are more common as you get older. We've noted earlier that as estrogen levels drop, the cells that line the vagina and urethra (the tube that leads from the bladder to the outside) change and the lining becomes thinner. Estrogen also helps lactobacilli grow. Lactobacilli are the bacteria that normally grows in the vagina and help keep it healthy. Lactobacilli makes the vaginal environment more acidic and suppresses the growth of other bacteria like E. coli, which can cause urinary tract infections. Lower levels of estrogen thus alter the vaginal environment, contributing to the increase in urinary tract infections.

Antibiotics

Antibiotics are used to treat urinary tract infections when they occur. Some women are prone to urinary tract infections after intercourse. During intercourse, bacteria are pushed into your urethra and the bladder. Usually, the bacteria are flushed out when you empty your bladder afterward. However, sometimes not all the bacteria are flushed out (especially in women who can't completely empty their bladder) and they multiply, causing a urinary tract infection. Those women who have urinary tract infections related to intercourse can take a dose of antibiotics after intercourse (after discussing with your physician) and prevent these infections.

Estrogen

It is controversial whether estrogen can help reduce the recurrence of urinary tract infections. Some studies have shown that estrogen decreases the likelihood of recurrent urinary tract infections while others have not. If you have problems with recurrent urinary tract infections, using estrogen does have potential risks and these should be carefully weighed against any benefits you may see (for more information on taking estrogen, refer to chapter 9).

Cranberry Juice

Cranberry juice has also been used to prevent recurrent urinary tract infections but the studies have been inconclusive as to its efficacy. Since the only downside to cranberry juice is its sugar content, if you like cranberry juice and are not allergic to it, go ahead and drink it. It may or may not help, but it wouldn't harm you.

BREAST CHANGES

Breast problems are most common in women between the ages of thirty-five and fifty-five.[24] Breast pain and tenderness, fibrocystic changes, formation of cysts, and breast cancer become more likely as the breasts change during perimenopause. The main concern that most women have with these breast changes is the possibility of breast cancer. Fortunately, most of the time, the suspected change is a benign condition and does not increase the risk of breast cancer. However, it is wise to be vigilant as the risk of breast cancer increases at this time.

For those in perimenopause, breast pain and tenderness is the most common breast symptom and is usually most prevalent the week or two before a period. Although you may have had some cyclical breast tenderness in the past, it can worsen during this phase. Although the discomfort is an annoyance for most women, for some it can be significant enough to interfere with their daily activities at work and at home.

Caffeine and chocolate can worsen breast pain in some women though it generally doesn't worsen the nodularity or lumpiness of the breast.[25] Birth control pills and hormone therapy with estrogen can also cause breast tenderness in some women. Lowering the dose of estrogen or switching to a different pill can sometimes help. Using a more supportive bra can also be helpful. Fortunately, most breast pain improves and usually resolves when you go through menopause and your estrogen levels decline (a positive side of menopause).

Vitamins and Medications for Breast Tenderness

Vitamins E, A, and B have been used to help with breast tenderness though no studies have shown them to be more effective than placebo.[26] Evening primrose oil has been found to be more effective than placebo in helping with breast pain in some studies.[27] It can also cause some nausea and may take a couple months to take effect. Furthermore, there is also some concern that it may cause some bleeding problems if taken in high doses or in women taking anticoagulants (medications to help thin the blood).

Other medications such as danazol, bromocriptine, GnRH agonists, and tamoxifen have been used with varying success, but can have significant side effects. Usually, only women who have extreme discomfort try these medications despite the potential side effects.

Other good news: your breasts become less dense as you get older and mammograms are better able to spot potential cancers.

HEADACHES

About 15 percent of all women suffer from migraine headaches.[28] Hormonal changes are an integral part of a woman's life cycle. Puberty, pregnancy, menopause, and the monthly menstrual cycles trigger natural changes in hormones. Hormonal forms of birth control and hormone therapy during menopause are other ways hormones can affect women.

Female hormones can promote migraine headaches. In children before puberty, there is no difference in migraines between boys and girls. However, adult women are three times more likely to suffer from migraines than adult men. For many women, migraines occur mainly or worsen around the time of their periods.[29]

Migraine headaches tend to be on one side of the head and pulsate. They may be worsened by physical activity, bright lights, and loud noises, and are associated with nausea. They usually last from four to seventy-two hours. About 20 percent of the migraine headaches are preceded by an "aura," usually visual, such as bright spots or halos around lights.[30]

Triggers of migraine headaches include:

- Stress or a drop in stress ("weekend" migraine)
- Hormonal changes
- Missing meals
- Deep sleep or sleeping too long
- Fatigue
- Foods (particularly chocolate, cheese, dairy products, fruit, alcohol —especially red wines—fried fatty foods, vegetables, tea, coffee, wheat, seafood)
- Chemical additives
- Certain medications
- Strong lights
- Weather changes
- Exertion
- High altitude

Hormones and Migraines

Migraines associated with periods seem to be triggered by a drop in estrogen levels. As women approach menopause, their migraines can either get better or worse as their hormones change. During perimenopause, there can be wide fluctuations in hormone levels, which may worsen migraine headaches. Migraine headaches peak when a woman is in her forties and fifties. After menopause, the female hormones level off at a new lower level and no longer fluctuate, leading to an improvement in migraines in roughly two-thirds of women.

The use of hormones during and after the perimenopausal period can also cause the migraines to improve or worsen. Changing the type of estrogen or progestin, or going from cyclic therapy (in which the progestin is given for ten to fourteen days of the month) to continuous therapy (where estrogen and progestin is given daily) can help with the headaches. Migraines do not seem to increase the risk of stroke in postmenopausal women so migraine headaches are not a contraindication to the use of hormones in these women.

Tension Headaches

Tension-type headaches affect 2 to 3 percent of the population. It is slightly more common in women than men and peaks around thirty to thirty-nine years of age. Tension headaches can coexist with migraine headaches and can also be precipitated by menstrual periods, although migraines tend to be more influenced by the hormonal changes of menopause, whereas tension headaches are more stress related.[31]

Tension headaches tend to be on both sides of the head, pressing or tightening in quality, and are generally not aggravated by physical activity. They are not associated with nausea or vomiting and usually not aggravated by bright lights or loud noises.

Triggers for tension headaches include:[32]

- Stress
- Mental tension
- Alcohol
- Weather changes
- Hormonal changes
- Fatigue

Treatment of migraine and tension headaches during perimenopause and menopause is no different than at other times. There have been suggestions that the use of hormones during perimenopause may help stabilize the hormone levels, thus lessening the severity of those tension headaches instigated by the widely fluctuating hormones, but this is not completely clear at this time.[33]

MEMORY AND COGNITIVE CHANGES

Many women complain about trouble remembering things, being forgetful, and having difficulties in concentrating as they begin menopause. "My memory just isn't what it used to be." "I'm so forgetful now." It is unclear if hormones play a direct role in these changes or if it is simply related to aging. As men age, their memory may also be affected. In women, hormones could be indirectly related to the extent that they cause hot flashes and night sweats, which may lead to poor sleep thus fostering these problems.

Mental Exercises

No magic pill exists that will help with memory or cognitive functioning, though there is some evidence that estrogen may help with some types of memory in postmenopausal women.[34] The best thing you can do, however, is to exercise both your mind and body. Playing games, reading, taking classes, and learning new hobbies or skills are several ways you can work your brain.

As many say—if you don't use it, you lose it. The more you engage your mind, the better it works. "But I'm too old to start learning new things," you might say. It's never too late to start stimulating your brain. Think of it as a chance to learn and do something you've always wanted to do, whether it's ballroom dancing, doing crossword puzzles, gardening, wood working, painting, or whatever catches your interest.

Physical Activity and the Brain

Physical activity also is good for the brain. Yet another reason for you to exercise. Being physically active increases blood flow and prevents the formation of plaques in the blood vessels that feed the brain. The better the blood flow, the more oxygen that goes to the brain. You don't have to join a gym to be more active. Go for a brisk walk. Park farther away at the store. Climb stairs instead of taking the elevator. Every little bit helps.

Stress Reduction

Stress reduction may also help keep your brain functioning better. High levels of stress hormones can impair memory. Chronic stress also contributes to depression and anxiety, which can interfere with memory. Learn relaxation techniques. Find other ways to relax whether you take a stroll outdoors, do some gardening, or play some music. Stay in close contact with friends and family and remain involved in activities that are meaningful to you.

Your Diet

Diet may have an impact on your brain. Studies show that lower fat diets in young and middle-aged adults may reduce the risk of Alzheimer's disease. Certain fruits and vegetables such as blueberries, strawberries, tomatoes, and broccoli are a good source for antioxidants and may also be beneficial. So your mom was right. Eat your fruits and veggies.

Antioxidant vitamins such as vitamins C and E may help protect the brain, though how much to take is unknown. Taking a general multivitamin is probably a reasonable way to supplement these vitamins at this time though it is probably better to get these vitamins and minerals through food.

Interestingly enough, drinking *small* amounts of alcohol (one to six drinks a week) may be helpful. Studies have shown that it lowered a person's risk for developing severe memory loss and Alzheimer's disease compared to nondrinkers and heavy drinkers.[35] However, there may be other differences in people who drink moderately from nondrinkers and heavy drinkers that may explain this finding. So don't start drinking just because you may think it may be helpful, because alcohol also has a number of harmful effects. Smoking, on the other hand, was found to be definitely harmful.[36]

FATIGUE

Some women complain of increased fatigue and decreased energy during perimenopause and blame it on hormonal changes. Hormones may play an indirect role in promoting the fatigue, as we've noted, by causing sleep disturbances. However, the most likely cause of the fatigue is the overwhelming number of tasks and activities that the modern woman has crammed in an average day.

And perimenopause and menopause is a time in your life when more and more things get piled on the plate: children (from infants to teenagers), work, home, spouse, parents, finances, and on and on. Eating habits worsen as you grab quick and easy foods to keep yourself going, exercise gets lost in the shuffle, and a good night's sleep becomes a luxury. Add to this the stress of trying to juggle all these things and you wonder why you aren't more tired.

Medical Problems That Can Cause Fatigue

But before you blame all on your lifestyle, you will want to make sure that there is no medical cause for the fatigue. Hypothyroidism, depression, and anemia are not uncommon causes of fatigue, especially in women.

Depression can be treated with counseling and/or medications (see chapter 4). During perimenopause, anemia can occur because of increased blood loss from heavier periods (please refer to chapter 3). Your physician can screen you for these problems.

Other medical problems can also cause fatigue and you may need further testing to determine if there are any other causes before assuming your loss of energy is purely the result of your hectic lifestyle or getting older.

Other symptoms such as changes in your sex drive and mood swings will be addressed in other chapters.

THE BOTTOM LINE

My wise mother once told me that you can't control what happens to you; you can only control how you react to a given situation. And it is the same with perimenopause and menopause. Like puberty, taxes, and death, it is inevitable and will eventually happen to all women. How each woman reacts depends on her strengths, history, coping mechanisms, and the perspective she takes.

CHAPTER 3

MY PERIODS HAVE CHANGED. SHOULD I WORRY?

Along with my forty-first birthday came my first sign of peri-menopause, irregular cycles. . . . Fortunately, my period is light and only lasts a few days and I have yet to experience a true "hot flash." So far my only complaint is the element of surprise I now experience and the lack of opportunity to plan for those monthly "occasions."

—Melissa B. Karasek

For most women, their monthly menstrual bleeding becomes a part of the natural rhythm of their lives. One of the first signs of peri-menopause can be a change in this rhythm. For some women, their periods will become irregular, sometimes coming three weeks apart, then skipping a month, and then coming two months later. For others, their periods may have always been twenty-eight days in the past, but are now every thirty-one or twenty-five days. Still others may notice that their periods are lighter, heavier, and/or shorter or longer in duration. There may or may not be a change in the consistency of the bleeding; some having more clotting while others have less. Not all women will experience this change in their cycles. They may continue to have their normal periods until they stop having them altogether, when they go through menopause.

Normal Menstrual Cycle

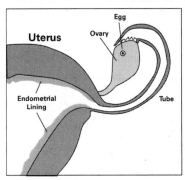

Figure 3.1. *At the beginning of your cycle, the endometrial lining is very thin and the egg is dormant in the ovary.*

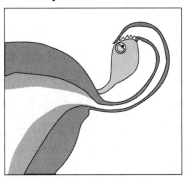

Figure 3.2. *Under the influence of your hormones, one egg starts to mature within a cyst. The endometrial lining thickens.*

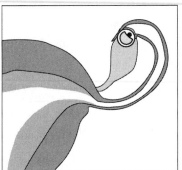

Figure 3.3. *The cyst on the ovary containing the egg gets larger (almost two centimeters) right before it pops to release the egg. The endometrial lining is thick at this time.*

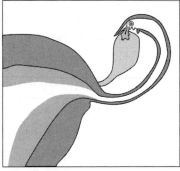

Figure 3.4. *When you ovulate, the cyst pops and releases the egg, which is then picked up by the fallopian tube.*

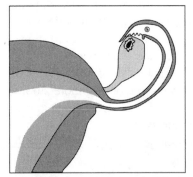

Figure 3.5. *The egg travels down the fallopian tube to the uterus. The shell of the cyst is then called the corpus luteum, which produces progesterone.*

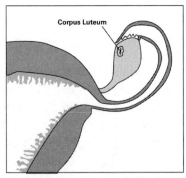

Figure 3.6. *If the egg is not fertilized, progesterone levels drop, and the lining of the uterus sloughs to form your menstrual flow.*

YOUR MENSTRUAL CYCLE

Your menstrual cycle is controlled by a complex interplay of hormones that come from the hypothalamus, pituitary gland, and ovary. An egg forms in a tiny cyst on your ovary. The cyst grows and grows, and in the middle of your cycle, it pops, releasing the egg. When the egg is released from the ovary, it is called ovulation. After you ovulate, there is a rise in the hormones estrogen and progesterone. The estrogen stimulates the lining of the uterus to thicken. Two weeks after the egg is released, the estrogen and progesterone levels drop and this signals the lining of the uterus to shed and be released. The lining of your uterus mixed with blood is what you see as your menstrual bleeding. This is the cycle that occurs month to month.

WHEN SHOULD YOU WORRY?

If changes in the menstrual cycle are normal during the perimenopausal period, then what should make you worry? Here are some potential warning signs that you need to bring to the attention of your physician:

- Bleeding between periods, even if it is only a very small amount
- Any bleeding after you have completely gone through menopause
- Significantly heavier bleeding than you normally experience
- Significantly longer periods than you normally experience
- Increased pain with your periods

What is normal? Normal menstrual cycles start every twenty-four to thirty-five days and last from two to seven days. However, some women have periods that may not quite fit this definition of "normal," with periods every thirty-eight days or lasting eight days. "Normal" is what you usually experience. The main thing to look for is any significant change in your own menstrual cycles.

What could these changes mean? Fortunately, most of the time, these changes are not a sign of something bad, but are caused by the changes in your hormones during this time. Instead of your hormones rising and falling in a smooth monthly cycle, they can become more erratic, leading to changes in your menstrual pattern. Since other problems can cause these menstrual changes, however, they need to be ruled out before it is assumed that hormones are responsible for the changes.

Other Causes of Menstrual Changes

When changes in your menstrual cycle occur, other conditions need to be ruled out before you can assume that the changes are related to hormones. These include:

- Dysfunctional uterine bleeding
- Pregnancy
- Polyps
- Fibroids
- Endometritis
- Adenomyosis
- Endometrial hyperplasia
- Cancer of the cervix, vagina, uterus, and fallopian tubes
- Bleeding disorders
- Thyroid problems
- Liver disease
- Medications

DYSFUNCTIONAL UTERINE BLEEDING

Dysfunctional uterine bleeding is defined as abnormal bleeding from the uterus that is not caused by a physical or medical problem. This diagnosis is made only after you have been evaluated and after other causes for bleeding have been eliminated. Dysfunctional uterine bleeding is usually caused by a change in the normal cycling of the hormones that comes from your body not releasing an egg or ovulating on a regular basis.

If your ovary does not release an egg, the hormones do not fall like they are supposed to and the lining of the uterus is not shed. The lining of the uterus continues to thicken and eventually gets so thick that a part of it sloughs off and comes out, which you see as bleeding. Then after a while, another part will slough off, and then another part. This happens without any pattern, leading to the irregular bleeding that you experience. The bleeding can also be severe and lead to anemia, and in rare cases the need for a blood transfusion.

Cause of Dysfunctional Uterine Bleeding

Dysfunctional uterine bleeding is very common during perimenopause because your ovaries release eggs more erratically at this time, instead of in their normal regular pattern. This is also commonly seen during puberty as the ovaries are developing and maturing. Since this is related to a change in the cycling of hormones, you may wonder if checking hormone levels would be useful to diagnose this condition. The short answer is, "No."

Your hormones fluctuate from day to day depending on where you are in your cycle, and the normal range is very wide. Even if a blood test is done during one cycle which shows that you did not ovulate during that cycle, you might ovulate with your next cycle. Regardless of the hormone levels, you are treated according to your symptoms, not your hormone numbers, so checking hormone levels won't change how you are treated.

Diagnosis of Dysfunctional Uterine Bleeding

Your physician will first talk to you and get more information about your bleeding. You will then be examined, looking for possible causes of bleeding such as cervical polyps, infections, or nongynecologic causes of bleeding (e.g., hemorrhoids). Sometimes, the bleeding may seem to be coming from the vagina, but is actually coming from another site such as the bladder or rectum.

The hematocrit, a blood test that checks for anemia, helps to determine how much blood has been lost. It can be difficult to tell how much blood has been lost by simply looking at the number of days of bleeding or pads used. Overestimation and underestimation of the amount of blood lost is not uncommon. Checking a hematocrit can help determine if you are losing more blood than your body can compensate for.

Blood tests, and other tests such as endometrial biopsy, ultrasound, sonohysterogram, and/or hysteroscopy, may also be performed to rule out other causes of bleeding such as polyps or fibroids (see below). If all the tests show no other physical or medical cause for the uterine bleeding, then you have dysfunctional uterine bleeding. Many times, dysfunctional uterine bleeding is called a "diagnosis of exclusion"; in other words, you have to exclude all other causes of bleeding to make this diagnosis.

Treatment of Dysfunctional Uterine Bleeding

Treatment of your bleeding problems depends on the cause of the bleeding as well as the degree that the bleeding is causing problems. If the bleeding is related to polyps, fibroids, thyroid problems, bleeding disorders, infection, liver disease, or medication, treating these problems can help with the bleeding (see below).

If the bleeding is not caused by a physical or medical problem (dysfunctional uterine bleeding), you have several options: watching and waiting, medical therapy, endometrial ablation, and hysterectomy.

If the bleeding is not very heavy or bothersome, you may choose just to live with it as long as you have ruled out any other serious causes for the bleeding. You will eventually go through menopause and the bleeding will generally stop (another positive side of menopause).

However, if the bleeding is causing anemia or having a significant impact on your life, you may want to consider other options:

- Iron
- Nonsteroidal anti-inflammatory drugs (NSAIDs)
- Birth control pills
- Progestins
- Endometrial ablation
- Hysterectomy

Iron

If you are bleeding very heavily, you could develop anemia. Anemia is a condition where there are low levels of red blood cells in the blood. Red blood cells carry the oxygen in your blood. If you bleed too much, your body cannot make enough red blood cells to compensate, which leads to anemia. Women with anemia may feel tired and without energy.

Iron is one of the main components of red blood cells. Most women take in enough iron in their diet to replace the amount lost in their menstrual blood. However, if women bleed too much, they may not have sufficient iron to make enough red blood cells to replace the ones lost. Taking in additional iron may be all that is necessary to resolve the anemia and no other treatment may be necessary. Some women develop constipation when they take frequent doses of iron. This can often be treated by increasing water intake, by increasing fiber intake, and by taking stool softeners.

Nonsteroidal Anti-Inflammatory Drugs (NSAIDs)

Prostaglandins are substances in the uterus that help regulate the bleeding that occurs with your periods. Nonsteroidal anti-inflammatory drugs (NSAIDs) such as ibuprofen and anaprox inhibit the formation of prosta-glandins and can decrease the amount of menstrual bleeding by about a third.[1] The main advantages are that NSAIDs need be taken only during your period to reduce bleeding and cramping. However, they can upset your stomach and can worsen certain conditions such as peptic ulcer disease.

Birth Control Pills

Birth control pills may help regulate cycles and decrease the amount of bleeding. (See chapter 7 for more information on the pill and its risks and benefits.)

Progestins

Progestins are progesterone-like hormones (see chapter 9 for more infor-mation about progestins). They can be given in two ways: cyclically or con-tinuously. When the progestins are given cyclically, it mimics the time before your period and causes the lining of your uterus to shed. This is helpful if you are having irregular bleeding due to your hormones not cycling normally when you don't ovulate. Progestins given continuously may make you have lighter periods or no periods at all. Side effects of progestins include irregular bleeding, weight gain, moodiness, bloating, and retention of fluid.

IUDs containing progestin can be placed in the uterus. The progestin acts directly on the lining of the uterus to make it thinner so that there is less lining to shed every month. Very little of the progestin is absorbed by the body so you have fewer side effects. (See chapter 7 for more informa-tion about IUDs.)

Endometrial Ablation

Endometrial ablation is a procedure by which the lining of the uterus (the endometrium) is destroyed. The lining is usually not completely destroyed, but enough is eliminated so that there is less lining to build up and less bleeding. The lining can be destroyed through a number of methods: laser, freezing, balloon, microwave, electrical coagulation, and resection. Regardless of the method used, the success rates are similar. About 70 to 90 percent of women have a satisfactory drop in menstrual bleeding.[2] Which method is used to destroy the lining of the uterus depends on your surgeon and what techniques he or she is comfortable using.

Endometrial ablation is done in outpatient surgery. The procedure usually starts with hysteroscopy and dilation and curettage (see below) to remove any polyps or fibroids and to scrape out the lining of the uterus so that the procedure is more effective. The lining is then destroyed. The recovery is similar to that of hysteroscopy. You tend to have more cramping after endometrial ablation, but the pain usually subsides within a couple of days.

Risks of Endometrial Ablation

In addition to the risks of hysteroscopy (see below), endometrial ablation carries additional risks. Part of the risk comes from the way the endometrial lining is destroyed. Using a laser, electrical energy, freezing, or heat can on rare occasions cause injury to surrounding organs such as the bowel or bladder. If this occurs, the damage can be serious and lead to the need for major surgery. Fortunately, this is very uncommon.

Other risks include the formation of scar tissue that can block the cervical canal. If this happens, when you are supposed to have a period, you will see little or no bleeding. The lining of your uterus and blood will be trapped inside the uterus. You will also have bad cramping because your uterus will be contracting to push the blood out but can't. If this happens, your surgeon will try to clear the blockage to let out the blood.

If the scar tissue blocks off just a small area, you may not have any immediate problems. One theoretical risk is that this may delay the diagnosis of endometrial (or uterine) cancer if it were to develop, since there would be no warning sign of bleeding. This is a theoretical risk, however. No studies have shown this to be a problem as yet.

Endometrial ablation is a relatively safe and effective alternative with a short recovery time. If you wish to have more children, though, you should not have this procedure done. Endometrial ablation may prevent you from getting pregnant and if you do get pregnant, it may potentially cause miscarriage or affect the ability of the pregnancy to grow normally. If you have an endometrial ablation, you will still need birth control however, since you may still be able to get pregnant.

Hysterectomy

Hysterectomy is a surgery that removes the uterus (which does not neces-sarily involve removing the ovaries). Removing the uterus will definitely stop the bleeding problem, but has the most risks. Hysterectomy is usually used as the last resort to treat dysfunctional uterine bleeding and only if there are significant problems such as severe anemia as a result of it. Hysterectomy eliminates any possibility of getting pregnant, which may be a good or bad thing, depending on whether or not you have finished having children.

Hysterectomy can be done in four ways: abdominal hysterectomy, vaginal hysterectomy, laparoscopic-assisted vaginal hysterectomy, and laparoscopic hysterectomy. Which approach is used depends on a number of factors that will be determined by your surgeon in communication with you.

Abdominal Hysterectomy

A cut is made on your abdomen, either a "bikini cut" like most women get with a Cesarean section or a vertical cut (a cut that goes up and down in the middle). Which type of cut is used depends on the size of the uterus and the reason for the hysterectomy. A vertical cut allows the surgeon to make a bigger opening, which is important if there are large fibroids or cancer.

After the surgery, you usually stay in the hospital for several days to recover. Once you get home, the first week or two are the most uncomfortable. Getting in and out of bed is very painful because it hurts to use your stomach muscles. It takes about six weeks to recover completely from this surgery.

Vaginal Hysterectomy

With a vaginal hysterectomy, the uterus is removed through the vagina. The recovery is much less painful and quicker because there is no cut on the stomach. In general, vaginal hysterectomy is technically more difficult to perform because there is less room and visibility. If there is not enough room or your uterus does not come down very well, your surgeon may not be able to perform a vaginal hysterectomy safely. Women who have never had a vaginal delivery, or who have never been pregnant, tend to have less room, which makes this approach more difficult.

One potential downside to this approach is that the ovaries may not be safely removed. The ovaries may be difficult to see and remove because of their location deep in the pelvis. Sometimes, the ovaries are easy to find and remove, but many times, they are too far away. So if a vaginal hysterectomy is performed, there is no guarantee that the ovaries could also be removed. (Later, we will discuss reasons why you would want or not want your ovaries removed.)

Most women stay in the hospital for one night after vaginal hysterectomy. They are up and moving quicker and experience less pain after surgery than those who opt for an abdominal or laparoscopic-assisted vaginal hysterectomy. Recovery from vaginal hysterectomy can take up to six weeks, but most women are doing well before that time.

Laparoscopic-Assisted Vaginal Hysterectomy

Laparoscopic-assisted vaginal hysterectomy uses laparoscopy (as described below) to help free the uterus from the ligaments holding it in the pelvis so that it can be removed vaginally. It is usually done when there is doubt that the hysterectomy can be done safely through only a vaginal approach. It avoids having to go through an abdominal hysterectomy with its larger cut on the abdomen.

Laparoscopy is a procedure where a laparoscope, a small telescope-type instrument, is placed through your belly button into the abdomen. Two other small cuts (about half an inch long) are made lower and to the sides through which other instruments are placed to staple, cut, and cauterize in order to detach the uterus.

The main advantages of this approach include: (1) Being able to examine the inside of the pelvis to make sure there is no scar tissue around the uterus. Scar tissue can attach the uterus to vital structures such as the bowel. If this happens, it can be difficult to see it during a vaginal hysterectomy, increasing the risk of damage to the bowel. Laparoscopy allows the surgeon to see if there is scar tissue and if there is, cut it so that the uterus is free. (2) Freeing up the uterus enough so that it can be removed vaginally. (3) Guaranteeing that the ovaries can be removed if desired. (4) Decreasing recovery time: recovery time in the hospital is usually overnight. The recovery and discomfort after surgery is generally worse than a vaginal hysterectomy but better than an abdominal hysterectomy.

Laparoscopic Hysterectomy

Laparoscopic hysterectomy removes the uterus completely with a laparoscope. The laparoscope is placed through the belly button into the abdomen. Two or three other small cuts are made below the belly button through which other instruments are placed to completely free the uterus. The uterus is then cut into small pieces to be able to remove it. The cervix is usually left behind.

This surgery is done mainly in women for whom vaginal hysterectomy and laparoscopic-assisted vaginal hysterectomy are not options. It is the least common type of hysterectomy performed and not all gynecologic surgeons know how to perform this procedure. There are a number of limitations to this procedure, however. For example, the uterus has to be cut into pieces for removal, and it must be determined beforehand that there is no uterine cancer. Cutting a uterus that had cancer could spread the cancer cells.

The main advantage of this approach is the shorter recovery time and decreased pain than after surgery from an abdominal hysterectomy. One night in the hospital is typical after a laparoscopic hysterectomy.

Limitations after any hysterectomy include no heavy lifting and pelvic rest: no tampons, douching, or intercourse for six weeks. There are also temporary restrictions against tub baths and swimming. If you require narcotics for pain control, you should not drive because narcotics, like alcohol, can affect your judgment. The main things to watch for after this surgery are signs of infection including fever, chills, increasing pain, and redness around or pus coming from your incision, if you have one. The pain should ease day by day, not worsen. If you have any of these problems, you should contact your surgeon immediately.

Risks of Hysterectomy

Hysterectomy is major surgery and as such has a number of risks including bleeding; infection; injury to other organs, such as your bowels, bladder, and ureters (the tubes connecting the kidney to the bladder); and blood clots in your legs. These risks and others will be reviewed when you discuss hysterectomy with your surgeon.

If Your Uterus Is Removed, Should the Ovaries Go, Too?

Your ovaries may or may not be removed at the time of hysterectomy done for dysfunctional uterine bleeding or any other reason. If your ovaries are removed, you will also go through menopause. If your ovaries are not removed, they will generally continue to produce hormones. So you would continue to have the same cyclical hormonal symptoms you had before, such as PMS, ovulation discomfort, and menstrual headaches, but no monthly bleeding to tell you where you are in your cycle. A number of factors will go into your decision to keep or remove your ovaries at the time of your hysterectomy, including your age and family or personal history of breast, ovarian, uterine, or colon cancer.

Your ovaries not only produce the female hormones estrogen and progesterone, but they are also a major source of testosterone in your body. Testosterone is mainly considered to be a "male" hormone, but it plays a role in a your sex drive, bone health, muscle strength, and general sense of well-being. Your testosterone levels decline during perimenopause, and continue to diminish more gradually for years after menopause. If your ovaries are removed, you also remove a major source of testosterone. If you have problems related to the drop in testosterone, you can take testosterone, but how much a woman needs is unclear and male hormone side effects such as hair growth, acne, oily skin, and deepening of the voice may occur.

The main advantages of removing your ovaries are that you will significantly decrease the chance that you will have ovarian cancer and will eliminate the need for future surgery for other potential ovarian problems later in life such as benign growths or painful cysts. Removing the ovaries reduces the chance of ovarian cancer, though it doesn't completely eliminate it.

An ovarian or peritoneal cancer (which looks and acts like an ovarian cancer) can arise even after both ovaries have been removed. This can occur because a tiny amount of ovarian tissue can be left behind. There is a thin layer of tissue that covers the pelvic and abdominal cavities called the peritoneum. This tissue can rarely give rise to peritoneal cancers which look, act, and spread just like ovarian cancers.

The advantages have to be weighed against these disadvantages:

- The possible need for more extensive surgery to remove the ovaries. Sometimes the ovaries can't be removed during vaginal hysterectomy. If that is the case, do you opt for the more involved laparoscopic-assisted vaginal hysterectomy just to remove the ovaries?
- Surgical menopause, which is more intense than natural menopause.
- The loss of testosterone, which may have a negative impact on libido, bone health, muscle strength, and general sense of well-being as noted above.

Other factors may also come into play. If you have a strong family history of ovarian, uterine, colon, or breast cancer, you may decide to remove your ovaries because these types of cancers tend to run in families. Having a strong family history of any of these cancers may, in fact, put you at increased risk of having ovarian cancer.

Your age is also important. If you have already gone through menopause, you don't need to worry as much about the symptoms of surgical menopause. Testosterone production may still be an issue, but production of this hormone would be declining at this time. If you are younger, you may be more apt to keep your ovaries because you have more years of ovarian function left and surgical menopause at a younger age is more intense. You will need to carefully discuss the pros and cons of removing your ovaries with your gynecologist to reach the right decision for you.

PREGNANCY

Because a woman's fertility significantly decreases in her forties, contraceptive use also decreases. Even a large decrease in fertility, however, still leaves open a window for these women to conceive. Because the likelihood of pregnancy is low in perimenopausal women, sometimes this possibility is overlooked. Remember that the two age groups with the highest number of unplanned pregnancies are teenagers and women over forty.

Bleeding can occur in normal pregnancies due to bleeding caused by implantation of the embryo. As the embryo attaches to the lining of the uterus, it can cause some bleeding. Bleeding can also be a sign of miscarriage or of an ectopic pregnancy (a pregnancy outside of the uterus). Even if a woman has had her tubes tied, there is a chance that an opening has formed, allowing conception to occur. If this has happened, there is a higher chance of an ectopic pregnancy. A pregnancy test is usually all that is needed to rule out this possibility. It is also important to remember that contraception should be used until a woman is clearly in menopause.

ENDOMETRIAL POLYPS

Endometrial polyps are growths in the uterine cavity that are generally benign. They can cause problems such as heavier periods as well as bleeding or spotting between periods. They may also cause cramping.

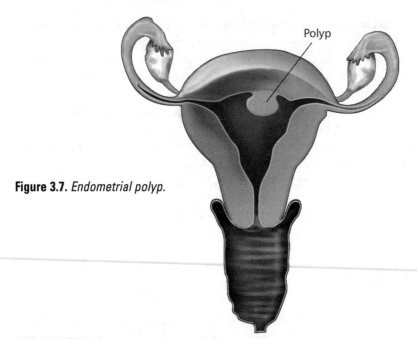

Polyp

Figure 3.7. *Endometrial polyp.*

Sometimes, polyps can make it harder to get pregnant by interfering with implantation of the embryo.

The endometrial polyp is made up of tissue from the lining of the uterus (also called the endometrium) that has grown out and sticks up from the lining. Polyps can come in different shapes and sizes. A polyp can look like a low mound rising out of the lining of the uterus. Or it can look like a lollipop with a ball of tissue connected by a thin stalk to the lining of the uterus (see figure 3.7). Polyps are soft and squishy, with the consistency of fat.

Most of the time, polyps are benign—not cancerous. But sometimes, a polyp may be hyperplastic or cancerous. The only way to tell this is to have the polyp removed and then evaluated by a pathologist, a medical doctor who specializes in examining tissues under the microscope.

Polyps can also arise from the cervical canal, forming endocervical polyps. These polyps can often be seen at the opening of the cervix and are usually benign.

How Do I Find Out If There Is a Polyp?

There are three tests that may be done to see if you have a polyp: pelvic ultrasound, sonohysterogram (or saline infusion sonography), and hysteroscopy.

Pelvic Ultrasound

Ultrasound uses sound waves to look inside the pelvis. The ultrasound can be done by placing the transducer—the part of the ultrasound machine that sends out and receives the sound waves—on your abdomen or in your vagina. The vaginal transducer is a wand a little thicker than your thumb. Transvaginal ultrasound, which is done by placing the transducer in the vagina, is usually a more accurate way of evaluating the uterus and ovaries.

The pictures obtained by ultrasound are grainy, black-and-white images. Ultrasound is good for looking at the lining of the uterus to see if it is abnormally thickened and at picking up fibroids (see below) and growths on your ovaries. A pelvic ultrasound can sometimes detect polyps, but generally it is not good at finding polyps in the uterus because polyps are usually the same consistency as the lining of the uterus and therefore cannot easily be distinguished from it. Ultrasound is like watching television with poor reception. You have an idea of what is there, but cannot tell exactly what it is.

Ultrasound uses sound waves, not x-rays, so there is no exposure to radiation and is safe. Transvaginal ultrasound can be a little uncomfortable for women who have never had vaginal intercourse or who are many years after menopause and are not currently having vaginal intercourse.

Sonohysterogram (Saline Infusion Sonography)

Sonohysterogram, also known as saline infusion sonography, is a procedure in which a small flexible plastic tube called a catheter is placed inside the uterus. The catheter is thinner than a pencil lead. Sonohysterogram is good at finding polyps or fibroids that are growing into the uterine cavity. This procedure is performed either in the office or radiology department. Sono-hysterogram may cause some cramping, though usually it is not as bad as the cramping caused by endometrial biopsy. Taking some ibuprofen before the procedure can help (if you are not allergic to it, discuss this possibility with your physician first). The procedure is ideally scheduled the week after your period because the lining to your uterus is thinnest at that time.

Before this procedure, a pregnancy test is usually done to rule out a pregnancy. A speculum is placed in the vagina, similar to when a Pap smear is done. The cervix is cleaned with betadine, an iodine solution (let your physician know if you are allergic to iodine). The catheter is threaded through the cervical canal into the uterus and the speculum is removed.

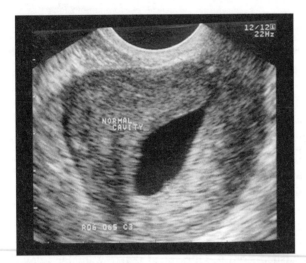

Figure 3.8. *Normal sonohysterogram.*

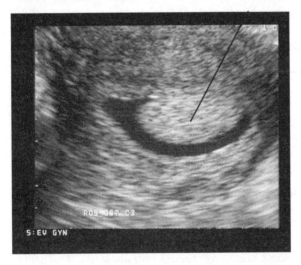

Figure 3.9. *Polyp seen on a sonohystero-gram.*

The transducer for the transvaginal ultrasound is placed in the vagina. A transvaginal ultrasound is then done while fluid is slowly pushed through the catheter into the uterus with a syringe. The fluid fills the uterine cavity, outlining the lining of the uterus. The lining of the uterus appears white on ultrasound while the fluid is black. If there is a polyp, it usually appears as a white ball or mound outlined by the black fluid (see figures 3.8 and 3.9).

After the sonohysterogram, you may have some spotting. You may be told to refrain from vaginal intercourse, douching, tampon use, and tub baths for several days after the procedure. The main thing to look for is increasing pain, discharge, and/or fever that could be a sign of infection.

Other possible problems that are very uncommon include pelvic infection, uterine perforation (the catheter may go through the wall of the uterus), and vagal response (where you feel nauseated, weak, light-headed, sweaty, and as if you are about to pass out).

Sometimes, the procedure is unsuccessful. If you have a very narrow cervical canal or there is a sharp turn, the catheter may not be able to be passed into the uterus. At times, the fluid does not stay in the uterus long enough to get a good view of the lining. And sometimes, a good view cannot be obtained through ultrasound, even with the fluid in place, because of the position of the uterus. There can be shadowing that can obscure the view, so things can be missed. Other times, it may look like there is something abnormal when there really isn't. If this happens, your physician will discuss other options to evaluate the inside of your uterus, such as hysteroscopy. But overall, the findings are very accurate, especially when done by someone experienced with this procedure and interpreted by a specialist.

Office Hysteroscopy

Hysteroscopy is a procedure by which a small, telescope-type instrument called the hysteroscope is placed inside the uterus. Hysteroscopy allows the physician to see clearly inside of the uterus. This procedure can be done in the office or through outpatient surgery. Office hysteroscopy is mainly used to look inside of the uterus to see if there is a problem. Since office hysteroscopy gives similar information to the sonohysterogram, usually one or the other is done to evaluate the inside of the uterus. Each has its advantages and the decision of which diagnostic tool is used is usually determined by the expertise of your physician.

With an office hysteroscopy, the surgeon can take a small biopsy if needed, but normally cannot remove polyps or fibroids. If done in the operating room, the surgeon uses a larger hysteroscope that can both determine if there is a problem and treat the problem immediately (such as removing a polyp). However, this procedure causes more pain and requires anesthesia, whereas office hysteroscopy often does not require any anesthesia.

The office hysteroscope is very small, about 3 mm in diameter. The hysteroscope has a camera attached to one end so the physician can see what is inside your uterus on a monitor. As with a sonohysterogram, an office hysteroscopy may cause some cramping, although it is usually not as

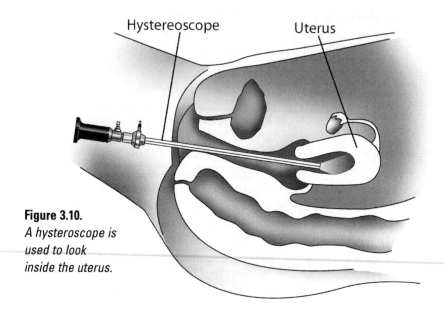

Hystereoscope   Uterus

Figure 3.10.
*A hysteroscope is
used to look
inside the uterus.*

bad as the cramping caused by endometrial biopsy. If recommended by your physician, taking some ibuprofen before the procedure can help. Again, the procedure is ideally scheduled the week after your period because the lining to your uterus is thinnest at that time.

The cervix is cleaned with betadine soap solution. An instrument called a single tooth tenaculum, as noted earlier, is used to grasp your cervix to stabilize it. This usually causes some cramping. Some physicians will sometimes use lidocaine to numb the cervix to reduce the cramping you may feel.

The hysteroscope is threaded through the cervical canal into the uterus. A gas is pumped through the hysteroscope into the uterus to open the uterus up like a balloon to allow the lining of the uterine cavity to be clearly seen. The physician will look throughout the uterine cavity and may take a biopsy.

After the hysteroscopy, you may have some spotting. You may be told to refrain from vaginal intercourse, douching, tampon use, and tub baths for several days after the procedure. You should watch for increasing pain, discharge, and/or fever that could be a sign of infection. As described earlier, other possible problems including uterine perforation and vagal response, are uncommon.

Sometimes an office hysteroscopy is unclear. Blood can obscure polyps or other problems. The gas may leak out so that the lining of the uterus cannot be blown open. The other downside is that if a polyp or fibroid is seen, you would then have to be scheduled for another procedure to remove it.

Treatment of Polyps: Hysteroscopy in the Operating Room

Some physicians prefer to perform hysteroscopy in the operating room because if a polyp or fibroid is discovered, it can be removed at that time. The patient also experiences less pain because of the anesthesia she receives. Diagnostic hysteroscopy and operative hysteroscopy are the two types of hysteroscopy done in this setting. Diagnostic hysteroscopy is similar to office hysteroscopy whereby the hysteroscope is placed inside the uterus to see if there are any visible problems. Operative hysteroscopy adds instruments to cut, freeze, or burn as needed to take care of a given problem.

Hysteroscopy is done in the operating room if there are findings on the sonohysterogram or office hysteroscopy (such as a polyp that need to be removed), or if the office diagnostic procedures were unsuccessful for whatever reason and the inside of the uterus needs to be further evaluated.

Fluid is usually used to blow up the uterus when hysteroscopy is done in the operating room. The use of fluid not only opens up the uterine cavity, but it also washes blood away, allowing for better visualization. Polyps are also sometimes easier to identify when floating in the fluid.

What Happens during Hysteroscopy

After you're asleep, the surgeon will dilate your cervix and place the hysteroscope in your uterus. What the surgeon finds determines what will be done next. Usually before the procedure your surgeon will have done an evaluation and have a pretty good idea of what to expect. The operating hysteroscope is about one centimeter in diameter.

Generally a wire loop with electricity running through it is used to cut, cauterize, or destroy any abnormalities inside of the uterus. Polyps and small fibroids can be cut out and removed. Or larger fibroids can be vaporized by electrical energy or by laser. Once the polyp or fibroid is removed, the lining of the uterus is scraped out. All of this tissue is sent to the pathology lab to be evaluated. The hysteroscopy can take anywhere from thirty minutes to a couple of hours to complete, depending on how much needs to be done.

After Hysteroscopy

Mild cramping and minor bleeding is not uncommon for several days after the procedure. Limitations after the procedure are mainly pelvic rest: no tampons, douching, or intercourse for one to two weeks. Tub baths and swimming are also usually restricted for that time. If you require narcotics for pain control, you should not drive. As noted earlier, narcotics, like alcohol, can affect your judgment. Generally, most women are able to return to work within a week.

The main things to watch for after this surgery are signs of infection including fever, chills, increasing pain, and foul-smelling discharge. The pain should lessen each day, not get worse. If you have heavy bleeding, especially if you are soaking through a pad or more in an hour, you should call your surgeon.

Risks of Hysteroscopy

Risks of hysteroscopy include infection, bleeding, uterine perforation (in which an instrument goes through the wall of the uterus), and Asherman's syndrome (scar tissue forms inside the uterus, which can make it difficult to get pregnant). Fortunately, the more serious complications are very uncommon. Complications are less common when hysteroscopy is performed by a surgeon who has done many of these procedures.

Removing the polyp usually ends the bleeding problem, though not always. While polyps can cause the bleeding problems, the bleeding instead could be caused by fluctuating hormone levels and the polyp may be a coincidental finding. Regardless, the polyp needs to be removed so that it can be evaluated. If the bleeding problems continue after removal of the polyp, then other treatment options may be tried.

FIBROIDS

Fibroids or leiomyomas are common benign growths in the uterus. They arise from the smooth muscle cells in the wall of the uterus, unlike polyps, which arise from the tissue that lines the inside of the uterus. Fibroids can grow anywhere in the uterus, from the inside lining, to deep in the wall, or on the outer surface, whereas endometrial polyps only grow inside the uterine cavity. About a quarter of all women have fibroids. They are more

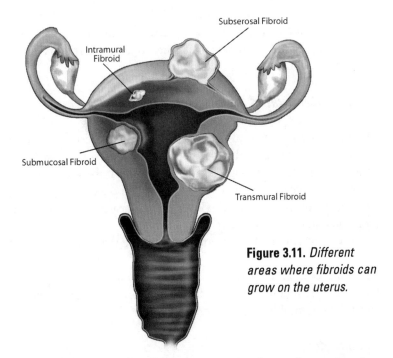

Figure 3.11. *Different areas where fibroids can grow on the uterus.*

common in African American women. They are hard, round growths, similar in consistency to cartilage. Most women who have fibroids have no problems with them.

Fibroids can grow in different parts of the uterus. If the fibroid is on the surface of the uterus, it is called a subserosal fibroid. Intramural fibroids grow inside the wall of the uterus, while submucosal fibroids grow in the uterine cavity. Transmural fibroids grow all the way through the full thickness of the uterine wall (see figure 3.11).

Fibroids cause problems mainly if they get very large and cause pelvic discomfort or pressure. They can also grow into the uterine cavity and result in heavier periods. They can also sometimes inhibit fertility. Fibroids do not need to be removed unless they are causing problems. In women over forty, there is a rare chance that the fibroid is not benign. This cancer known as leiomyosarcoma is very rare.

A submucosal fibroid can be removed by hysteroscopy. Most of the time, this is all that is needed to control the heavy bleeding that can be caused by a submucosal fibroid. Occasionally, the fibroid may not be completely removed and grow back, or another fibroid may grow and the bleeding problems may recur.

If the fibroid is on the outside of the uterus, or it goes all the way from the inside of the uterus to the outer surface of the uterus, or it is too large to remove with a hysteroscope, other treatment options are available including myomectomy or hysterectomy.

Surgical Removal of Fibroids (Myomectomy)

Myomectomy is a type of surgery in which just the fibroids are removed but the uterus is left in place. Myomectomy can be done by hysteroscopy as described above, through a larger incision on the abdomen, or through laparoscopy. Typically, larger fibroids are removed through a larger incision or cut on the abdomen. Generally, laparoscopic surgery causes less pain and entails a shorter recovery.

Myomectomy is done if you want to save the uterus, mainly for pregnancy. The risks of and recovery from myomectomy when done through a larger incision on the abdomen are similar to hysterectomy. The main disadvantage of myomectomy is that the fibroids can grow back, possibly causing more problems in the future.

Hysterectomy

Hysterectomy, as noted above, is a surgery that removes the uterus (which does not necessarily involve removing the ovaries). Removing the uterus will permanently resolve the fibroid problem and relieve its symptoms of bleeding and/or pressure. A hysterectomy is the final option. It is guaranteed to stop your bleeding and your periods, and prevent the recurrence of the fibroids. However, hysterectomy entails more risks, pain, and recovery time than hysteroscopy and eliminates any possibility of getting pregnant. (See above for more information about hysterectomy.)

GnRH (Gonadotropin-Releasing Hormone) Agonists

GnRH (Gonadotropin-Releasing Hormone) agonists such as Depo-Lupron are medicines that basically shut down the ovaries, leading to a drop in estrogen levels and temporary menopause. The lack of estrogen brought about by GnRH agonists leads to temporary shrinking of the fibroids. The main role of these medications is to stop the bleeding to help a woman build up her blood before surgery or to shrink the fibroids so they can be removed easier during surgery. Once the GnRH agonist is discontinued, the fibroids grow back to their original size. Because the use of this medication is limited to not more than a year, it is not a long-term solution for fibroids.

Most women will have a significant drop in their bleeding or no bleeding while on this medicine. However, they will experience the same feelings they would have when going through menopause such as hot flashes, night sweats, vaginal dryness, etc. Generally, GnRH agonists are not used for more than six to twelve months because of the concern about bone loss.

Depo-Lupron is the most common GnRH agonist used and is given as a shot, either once a month or every three months. GnRH agonists can significantly decrease the amount of bleeding so that if a woman is significantly anemic, it will allow her to build up her blood level. If she is planning to have a hysterectomy, this may decrease the likelihood that she may need a blood transfusion during or after surgery. GnRH agonists are also useful to help control bleeding in a woman about to go through menopause. If the bleeding problems can be controlled for a while, this may get a woman closer to menopause when she will no longer have any menstrual bleeding.

The main disadvantages of GnRH agonists are the menopausal side effects and potential for causing bone loss because of the loss of estrogen. Progestin with or without estrogen is sometimes used as "add-back" therapy, whereby hormones are added back to these women to help decrease these side effects. However, because of the above concerns, GnRH agonists are generally not considered a long-term option.

Uterine Artery Embolization

Another relatively newer treatment option is uterine artery embolization. A radiologist guides a catheter (a thin tube) into the main arteries that feed the uterus. Tiny coils are placed through the catheter to block these arteries. This inhibits blood flow to the uterus, causing fibroids to shrink considerably because of the lack of blood. Uterine artery embolization is quite uncomfortable, however.

Pregnancy is not recommended after this procedure because the blood supply to the uterus has been diminished and may adversely affect a pregnancy. Complications of uterine artery embolization include hematoma (blood clot at the catheter insertion site); postembolization syndrome, which is characterized by fever, chills, malaise, and decreased appetite; pelvic infections; kidney failure; and in very rare cases, death. Sexual problems such as painful intercourse can sometimes occur after this procedure.[3] Fortunately, the likelihood of a serious complication is rare.

ENDOMETRIAL HYPERPLASIA

Endometrial hyperplasia is a condition in which there is an overgrowth of the lining of the uterus. Normally, estrogen causes the lining of the uterus to grow and thicken and progesterone keeps the lining from getting too thick. A drop in the progesterone level at the end of the cycle is the trigger that sheds the lining of the uterus. Endometrial hyperplasia results when the uterine lining is exposed to too much estrogen and not enough progesterone.

Endometrial hyperplasia manifests as abnormal bleeding such as heavier periods, spotting or bleeding between periods, or any bleeding after menopause. Usually, it doesn't cause any pain or other symptoms.

The main concern is that endometrial hyperplasia can lead to endometrial cancer if untreated. Endometrial hyperplasia is divided into different categories depending on its appearance, which is also related to its risk of progression to cancer. With hyperplasia, the cells are overly abundant, but still look normal. Simple and complex hyperplasia refers to the degree of overgrowth. When the cells become abnormal looking, the hyperplasia is labeled as having "atypia." In other words, the cells are atypical in appearance, but not cancerous.

Risk of Types of Endometrial Hyperplasia Progressing to Endometrial Cancer[4]

Type of Hyperplasia	Progression to Cancer
Simple hyperplasia without atypia	1%
Complex hyperplasia without atypia	3%
Simple hyperplasia with atypia	8%
Complex hyperplasia with atypia	29%

To find out if you have endometrial hyperplasia, a sample of the uterine lining needs to be obtained. This can be done in the office by endometrial biopsy or in the operating room by a dilation and curettage (D&C). Usually, an endometrial biopsy is done first because it is safer than a D&C, which is a surgical procedure. If an endometrial biopsy is unsuccessful or inadequate, then a D&C is done.

Endometrial Biopsy

Endometrial biopsy is used to obtain a tissue sample of the lining of the uterus. This tissue sample is sent to a lab where a pathologist examines it under a microscope. By looking at this tissue, the pathologist can determine if it is normal, hyperplastic, or cancerous. Sometimes a definitive answer cannot be made and further tests may be needed.

Endometrial biopsy is performed in the office setting. It can be a fairly uncomfortable procedure, depending on: how much manipulation is necessary, if you have had a vaginal delivery, the sensitivity of your cervix and uterus, and your own level of pain tolerance. Ideally, you should not be having your period when you are having this procedure performed because a good specimen may not be obtained. You may take some ibuprofen (if you're not allergic to it) beforehand, which will help lessen the cramping. If you have a low tolerance to pain, your physician may prescribe stronger pain medicines to take before the procedure, but you will need to have someone drive you home.

In the office, a pregnancy test is usually done before the procedure to rule out a pregnancy. If you are pregnant and have the endometrial biopsy done, there is a good chance that it will disrupt the pregnancy and cause a miscarriage.

How Endometrial Biopsy Is Done

A speculum is placed in the vagina, similar to when a Pap smear is done. The cervix is cleaned with betadine soap solution. If you have an allergy to iodine, then a different cleaning solution will be used. A single-tooth tenaculum may be used to grasp your cervix to stabilize it. This usually causes some cramping.

The pipelle, a thin flexible plastic tube about 3 mm in diameter, is threaded through the cervical canal into the uterus. Suction is created inside of the tube by pulling out a plunger from the tube or by using a syringe. The pipelle is then rotated as it is moved inside of the uterus and the suction pulls tissue from the lining into the pipelle. This part lasts for half a minute to a minute and is what causes most of the pain. Once the sample is obtained, the pipelle and the single-tooth tenaculum are removed. The cramping usually subsides over the next couple of hours.

Sometimes, especially if you have never had a vaginal delivery or if it has been many years since you have gone through menopause, you may have what is called a stenotic os. A stenotic os is a condition where the cervical opening, called the cervical os, is very narrow. Your physician may try to dilate or open up the cervical opening enough to place the pipelle into the uterus. Some physicians will sometimes use lidocaine to numb the cervix to reduce the cramping you may feel. However, other physicians choose not to because they feel that the discomfort from the numbing is as bad or worse than the discomfort from dilating the cervix. The cervical opening may be too narrow and an endometrial biopsy may not be able to be done.

Side Effects of Endometrial Biopsy

After the biopsy, you will probably have some spotting. You may be told to refrain from vaginal intercourse, douching, tampon use, and tub baths for several days after the procedure. The main thing to be aware of is increasing pain, discharge, and/or fever, which could be signs of an infection.

Other uncommon problems associated with the procedure include vagal response (where you feel nauseated, weak, lightheaded, and sweaty, and as if you are about to pass out) and uterine perforation (where the pipelle goes through the wall of the uterus, very rare).

The results of the biopsy are usually back within one to two weeks. Sometimes, not enough tissue is obtained and a definitive answer cannot be given. If the endometrial biopsy is unable to be done or if the specimen is inadequate, D&C with or without a hysteroscopy is generally recommended.

Dilation and Curettage (D&C)

Dilation and curettage (D&C) is a procedure usually done as outpatient surgery. The cervix is dilated or opened up enough to put an instrument inside the uterus so that the lining can be scraped. The instrument is not sharp but relatively dull. The procedure is actually akin to scraping out melon seeds using a spoon.

The main purpose of this procedure is to get a good sampling of the lining of the uterus to see what is there. It is considered a "blind" procedure. The surgeon can't see what he or she is scraping; it's done by feel. D&C is a good procedure to rule out endometrial cancer and hyperplasia, but if a polyp is present, there is a chance that it may be missed and left inside.

D&C is similar to an endometrial biopsy in that they are both ways of getting a sample of the uterine lining.

The advantages of a D&C over endometrial biopsy include:

- The use of anesthesia to help with the discomfort
- The availability of specialized equipment if the cervix is very narrow to help open the cervix
- The possibility of removing other problems such as polyps, though this is not guaranteed

D&C is usually done *with hysteroscopy* to evaluate abnormal bleeding. In the past, before the advent of hysteroscopy, D&C by itself was performed to evaluate and treat women with abnormal bleeding. However, because hysteroscopy enables the surgeon to see inside the uterus and selectively remove any abnormality such as polyps, D&C is usually not done by itself anymore when evaluating a woman for bleeding problems.

The types of anesthesia used, risks involved, and recovery from D&C are similar to those of hysteroscopy.

Treatment of Endometrial Hyperplasia

Endometrial hyperplasia without atypia can be treated with progestins (compounds that act like progesterone) for three to six months. The progestins suppress the growth of endometrial cells, generally making the hyperplasia regress and turn back to normal. An endometrial biopsy is done at the end of that treatment to confirm the hyperplasia is gone.

If there is endometrial hyperplasia *with* atypia, treatment depends on whether you want to keep your uterus or not. Generally, the first choice of treatment is a hysterectomy to remove the uterus because of the significant chance (8 to 29 percent chance in one study[5]) that the hyperplasia will progress to cancer if untreated. The other concern is that there may already be cancer if the biopsy shows endometrial hyperplasia with atypia. However, if you still want to have children or have other significant medical problems that would make surgery risky, then you may be treated with progestins instead of a hysterectomy.

If you and your physician choose to treat endometrial hyperplasia with atypia using progestins, a more thorough sample of the lining of the uterus should be done by D&C to rule out cancer that may have been missed with the endometrial biopsy. Endometrial biopsy should be done on a periodic basis (some physicians suggest every six months) because there is a high chance that the endometrial hyperplasia will come back even after treatment. If you have a hysterectomy, you would not have to worry about recurrence and would be cured.

ENDOMETRIAL CANCER

Endometrial cancer is a cancer of the lining of the uterus. It is sometimes called uterine cancer. The American Cancer Society estimates that about forty thousand women will be diagnosed with uterine cancer each year in this country.[6] It is the most common gynecologic cancer in women. Fortunately, endometrial cancer is usually caught early because it causes abnormal uterine bleeding.

Endometrial cancer is found in less than 10 percent of women with abnormal bleeding during perimenopause but in about 25 percent of women who are postmenopausal.[7] Most of the time, the abnormal bleeding is not caused by cancer. But since cancer is such a serious problem, you want to make sure that a cancer is not missed before dismissing the bleeding problems as caused by hormonal changes related to perimenopause.

The risk factors for endometrial cancer include:

- Being overweight
- Having no children
- Late menopause
- Diabetes
- History of radiation therapy
- High blood pressure
- Using estrogen alone (without progestins) after menopause
- History of breast, ovarian, or colon cancer
- History of polycystic ovarian syndrome
- Tamoxifen use
- Family history of endometrial, breast, colon, or ovarian cancer

Many of these risk factors are related to higher estrogen levels which cause the endometrial cells to grow and grow. Eventually, they can start to change and become cancerous.

Endometrial cancer is usually diagnosed through an endometrial biopsy or D&C. A thickened endometrial lining as seen on pelvic ultrasound can sometimes be a sign of endometrial cancer and needs to be evaluated further with endometrial biopsy or D&C. Since it is usually caught early, hysterectomy is generally all that is needed. Moreover, cure rates are very high since endometrial cancer is generally caught early. Sometimes if the cancer has spread radiation therapy is needed.

ENDOMETRITIS

Endometritis is an infection of the lining of the uterus. It can be caused by sexually transmitted organisms such as gonorrhea or chlamydia, but can also be caused by other bacteria. Endometritis can result in abnormal or heavy bleeding and a dull, constant ache in the pelvis. Endometritis is diagnosed by an endometrial biopsy and culture. Antibiotics usually cure this problem.

ADENOMYOSIS

Adenomyosis is a condition in which part of the lining of the uterus (the endometrium) grows into the uterine walls. Adenomyosis is seen mostly in women over the age of thirty-five who have had children. Adenomyosis can lead to several problems including painful periods, heavier periods, and pain during intercourse deep in the pelvis. Unfortunately, a definite diagnosis of adenomyosis can be made only by looking at the uterus under a microscope after a hysterectomy. MRI (magnetic resonance imaging) and ultrasound can sometimes detect adenomyosis without surgery, but not reliably.

Laparoscopy cannot be used to diagnose adenomyosis because only the outside of the uterus is visible. The uterus may have a certain red and boggy appearance that can make your surgeon suspicious for adenomyosis, but the only way to see if it is truly there is to look at the uterus under a microscope.

If adenomyosis is suspected, it can be treated with nonsteroidal anti-inflammatory drugs (such as ibuprofen) and hormones such as birth control pills, progestins, and GnRH agonists. Hormonal treatment of adenomyosis can sometimes render it less active and less painful. However, if these measures fail, hysterectomy may be necessary. Many times after menopause, the symptoms improve or resolve themselves.

CERVICAL CANCER

Cancer of the cervix can first present itself as abnormal bleeding. The cancerous cervix is friable, raw, and bleeds more easily. The bleeding is sometimes first noticed after sexual intercourse. Pap smears screen for cervical cancer and usually catch changes on the cervix before they become cancerous. (See human papillomavirus in chapter 8.)

Cervical Dysplasia: Precursor to Cancer

These interim changes are called cervical dysplasia, which is a condition in which abnormal changes appear in the cervical cells. This is almost always caused by the human papilloma virus, which is generally spread by sexual contact. The virus gets into the cervical cells and changes them. Sometimes, if the cervical dysplasia is not treated (by freezing, lasering, or cutting out the abnormal cells), it can progress to cervical cancer. This progression from cervical dysplasia to cervical cancer usually takes several years. Regular Pap smears are recommended to discover these changes early.

Treatment of Cervical Cancer

Treatment of cervical cancer is either by a radical hysterectomy or radiation depending on how large the cancer is and how far it has spread. A radical hysterectomy involves removal of the uterus and tissues surrounding the uterus. Very tiny cancers of the cervix can sometimes be treated with a cone biopsy if a woman wishes to preserve her ability to get pregnant. A cone biopsy is an outpatient procedure in which a cone-shaped section of the cervix is removed along with the cancer. A cone biopsy is also done when cervical cancer is suspected to see if it is present or not.

VAGINAL CANCER

Cancer of the vagina is quite uncommon, but may also initially appear as vaginal bleeding. Many times, the Pap smear can detect vaginal dysplasia, which is the precursor to vaginal cancer and similar to cervical dysplasia. Vaginal cancer is treated by surgery and/or radiation depending on where the cancer is located, how large it is, and how far it has spread.

FALLOPIAN TUBE CANCER

Fallopian tube cancer is the rarest gynecologic cancer and can sometimes manifest as abnormal vaginal bleeding. It is treated with surgery and chemotherapy.

LIVER DISEASE

Women with severe liver disease such as cirrhosis are not able to produce adequate amounts of certain clotting factors. When these clotting factors decrease below a certain level, blood does not clot very well, which causes bleeding problems.

The liver also metabolizes or breaks down estrogen. When the liver disease is severe, it actually results in an increase in estrogen levels. The estrogen stimulates the uterine lining to grow, which may lead to endometrial hyperplasia and bleeding problems.

The liver may be damaged as a result of hepatitis or excessive alcohol consumption. Even two alcoholic drinks a day, which may not seem much, may eventually lead to liver problems in women. If the liver becomes severely damaged, these problems may progress and lead to death.

THYROID PROBLEMS

Thyroid problems can also cause changes in your menstrual cycle. The thyroid is responsible for regulating the body's metabolism. Hypothyroidism and hyperthyroidism can trigger changes in the menstrual cycle such as irregular or very heavy bleeding. (See chapter 12 for more information about thyroid problems.)

BLEEDING DISORDERS

The first sign of a bleeding disorder such as thrombocytopenic purpura (a condition where there is a decrease in blood platelets) can be heavier periods. Bleeding disorders may be due to a decrease in platelets, which are irregularly shaped disks that are about a third the size of a red blood cell and are essential in helping the blood clot. Bleeding problems may also derive from a deficiency of certain factors that help blood clot. A series of reactions occurs to make blood clot. A deficiency in one of the many factors involved in clotting can lead to bleeding problems.

Other signs of bleeding disorders are easy bruising, bleeding heavily after minor injuries or procedures, bleeding easily from the gums, and having relatives with bleeding disorders. Many times, people are unaware that they have a bleeding disorder because they feel that their problems are relatively minor and are normal for them or don't show up until they have had an accident or surgery, which makes their clotting problem obvious.

Bleeding disorders are usually diagnosed by doing blood tests. Treatment depends on the specific bleeding disorder.

MEDICATIONS

Hormones such as birth control pills and hormone replacement therapy, steroids, antiseizure medications, antidepressants, and anticoagulants, as well as the IUD, can all cause menstrual bleeding problems. Be sure your physician reviews your medications and any over-the-counter supplements you are taking. Some herbal products may also cause bleeding problems.

THE BOTTOM LINE

In summary, most changes in your periods during perimenopause are related to hormonal changes. But you need to be evaluated to make sure that nothing else is being missed before making this assumption. If there are problems causing these changes, they can be treated by a variety of methods, each of which has its advantages and disadvantages. You need to be in communication with your physician and work closely with him or her to determine what is right for you.

CHAPTER 4

WHAT'S WITH MY MOODS?

When it takes tremendous restraint from putting a bullet through your husband's head just because he is noisily eating a raw carrot stick, you know you are in menopause.

—Nancy Cavegn

M any women notice a change in their moods when they enter their thirties and forties. "This isn't me. I'm not like this." "I've always been a very level person. I don't know what's come over me." "I hear myself yelling and I know I shouldn't but I can't stop myself." "I find myself crying for no reason." Why does this happen? Is it a hormonal problem? Do you just have to live with it?

Worsening premenstrual syndrome (PMS) and depressive symptoms have been associated with perimenopause and menopause. Fortunately, for most women, the moodiness and irritability are a minor problem if they have this problem at all. Those who enjoy positive moods during perimenopause and menopause likely had positive moods before this transition (the most important factor) and are living with a partner, have low interpersonal stress, have a positive attitude toward aging, have work satisfaction, have fewer daily hassles, and have fewer major negative life events (such as divorce, death in the family, or major illness).[1]

Many women notice that the changes in their mood are worse the week or two before their periods. Premenstrual syndrome is defined as "the cyclical recurrence of physical, psychologic, or behavioral symptoms that appear after ovulation and resolve within a few days after the onset of menstruation."[2] PMS seems to worsen during perimenopause. This could be related to wider fluctuations in hormones and/or an increase in sensitivity to these hormonal changes. The good news is that once your periods end when you go through menopause, your PMS symptoms will also come to an end.

Some women may notice that they feel more depressed during perimenopause and menopause. The depression may be constant or change with their cycles. They may feel only a little "blue," or the symptoms may be much more severe and lead to thoughts of worthlessness or, in rare cases, even suicide. Some researchers feel that depression becomes more common in women during perimenopause, though this is still under debate. We will explore both PMS and depression in this chapter.

PREMENSTRUAL SYNDROME (PMS)

PMS may worsen during perimenopause. More than 150 different symptoms have been associated with PMS. The symptoms can be divided into mood or emotional symptoms and physical symptoms.

More common physical symptoms of premenstrual syndrome include:

- Bloating
- Fluid retention
- Weight gain
- Breast tenderness
- Lack of energy
- Acne
- Increased appetite

Mood symptoms of premenstrual syndrome include:

- Irritability
- Mood swings
- Anxiety
- Tension
- Depression

- Crying spells
- Short tempered, anger
- Poor concentration

Surveys estimate that 90 percent of women have experienced at least one premenstrual symptom. For most women the symptoms are mild and remain physical in nature, such as bloating or breast tenderness. About 30 percent in surveys say that their symptoms are "moderate" and 3 to 8 percent say they are "severe."[3] Severe symptoms can significantly impact a woman's life, affecting her relationships, work, and quality of life.

It is important to emphasize that with *pre*menstrual syndrome the symptoms should be present only during the week or two *before* the period. The symptoms should be absent for the rest of the cycle. Some women have ongoing problems that intensify the week or two before their periods. For example, if you have depression and it worsens before your period, that's not PMS. You have depression that worsens before your period.

HOW CAN YOU TELL IF YOU HAVE PMS?

No test is available that can diagnose PMS. Testing hormone levels is not helpful because women with PMS generally have normal levels of hormones. The way to see if you have PMS is to keep a diary of your symptoms. On a calendar, mark your periods. Grade your symptoms on a scale of 1 to 3, 1 being minimal symptoms, 2 being moderate symptoms, and 3 indicating severe symptoms. Plot your symptoms over three months and see if there is a pattern.

If you see that your symptoms are clustered in the week or two before your period and you are relatively symptom-free the other times, you have PMS. There is no minimum number of symptoms you must have in order to have PMS.

Many conditions can be exacerbated by the hormonal changes before your period: anxiety, depression, and headaches, to name a few. Some people refer to this as premenstrual magnification. Treating PMS or premenstrual magnification during the premenstrual period is similar, however.

PREMENSTRUAL DYSPHORIC DISORDER (PMDD)

Premenstrual dysphoric disorder or PMDD is a severe form of PMS. PMDD has much stricter criteria and the symptoms must be severe enough to interfere with relationships, social functioning, and quality of life.

To have PMDD the following criteria must be met:[4]

1. During most of the menstrual cycles in the past year you must have five or more of the following symptoms, one of which has to come from the first four on the list:

   - Severely depressed mood, feelings of hopelessness, or self deprecating thoughts (thinking very badly about yourself)
   - Significant anxiety, tension, and/or feelings of being "on edge" or "keyed up"
   - Severe mood swings (you may feel suddenly sad and tearful or very sensitive to rejection)
   - Persistent and marked anger, irritability, or increased conflicts with others
   - Decreased interest in usual activities (i.e., work, friends, hobbies)
   - Difficulty in concentrating
   - Fatigue, lack of energy
   - Major change in appetite, overeating, or food cravings
   - Insomnia or oversleeping
   - A feeling of being overwhelmed or out of control
   - Other physical symptoms such as breast tenderness or swelling, headaches, joint or muscle pain, bloating, or weight gain

   The symptoms are present during the week before your period starts, should begin to improve within a few days after the beginning of your period, and should be absent in the week after your period ends.

2. The symptoms must significantly interfere with work or school or with usual social activities and relationships with others.

3. The symptom is not an exacerbation of another disorder such as depression (to be discussed later), panic disorder, or personality disorder, although PMDD may be superimposed on any of these disorders.

4. The diagnosis must be confirmed by doing daily ratings of symptoms for at least two cycles with symptoms.

Care must be taken to ensure that the symptoms are not caused by other medical or psychiatric disorders that can mimic PMS or PMDD. Medical conditions such as hypothyroidism, anemia, hypoglycemia, and autoimmune disorders should be excluded. Depression and bipolar, anxiety, panic, and personality disorders, as well as drug and alcohol abuse, should be ruled out also.

Many of these other disorders may have an exacerbation of their symptoms during the premenstrual phase, making it seem like PMS. However, if you follow the symptoms closely, many times you will see that they are always present, just worse before your periods. When the underlying disorder is treated, many times what was thought to be premenstrual syndrome clears up, is controlled, or is significantly improved.

WHAT CAUSES PMS OR PMDD?

Numerous theories on the cause of PMS and PMDD (to be referred to collectively as PMS) have been proposed, but still there is no definitive answer for them. The current consensus is that the normal hormonal changes during the menstrual cycle are the trigger for these symptoms, *not* a hormonal imbalance as previously thought.[5] Personality disorders have also been eliminated as an explanation for the cause of these symptoms in the cases of PMS.

A rise in progesterone and estrogen occurs in the second half of the menstrual cycle. Suppressing these hormones has been shown to eliminate PMS symptoms. This can be done through medications such as GnRH agonists that temporarily shut down the ovaries, by removing both ovaries surgically, or by simply going through menopause. Somehow, the normal changes in hormones triggers something in some women that leads to PMS.

Evidence is accumulating that certain neurotransmitters (chemicals that let nerves communicate with each other) such as serotonin and gamma-amino butyric acid (GABA) may be involved in the symptoms of PMS. Perhaps the change in hormones causes an alteration in these neurotransmitters in some women that leads to PMS. There may also be a genetic component to PMS. Mothers who have PMS are more likely to have daughters who develop PMS. A twin also seems to be more likely to have severe PMS if the identical twin has it rather than in the case of a fraternal twin.[6]

Though the exact cause of PMS is still unclear, what is becoming more evident is that PMS is caused by actual changes in the body and is not something that's "just in your head."

TREATMENT OF PMS

Most women do not need any treatment for their PMS symptoms because their symptoms are minor. For women whose symptoms are more severe, treatment options are available. What a woman chooses to do depends on the severity of the symptoms and her perception of the treatment choices.

For example, a woman may have some irritability before her periods that is bothersome enough for her to want to try to improve it. She may choose to exercise and take calcium supplements, preferring not to use medications, since her symptoms are not that severe.

Even if a woman's symptoms are more severe, she may choose to use a "stepwise" approach, starting with lifestyle changes and supplements and progressing onto prescription medications if the initial measures fail. Other women with extremely severe symptoms may desire relief as quickly as possible and may wish to start with medications first.

Hundreds of treatments have been tried to alleviate symptoms of PMS. Some have been shown to help with all symptoms—physical and emotional—while others are helpful for only certain symptoms. Because of a large placebo response to treatment, many interventions that were initially thought to be effective were later shown not to be when studied more rigorously. We will review the treatments that currently have been proven to help.

Lifestyle Changes

Aerobic Exercise

Regular aerobic exercise may help with PMS. Studies that compare women who exercise with those who do not, show that exercisers have fewer PMS symptoms.[7] Aerobic exercise causes an increase in endorphins, which may help with moods. Aerobic exercise has numerous other health benefits and should be recommended for everyone. Unfortunately, during perimenopause, which is when PMS may worsen, many women become less and less active.

Dietary Changes

A number of dietary changes have been recommended to help reduce PMS symptoms including decreasing salt, sugar, alcohol, and caffeine while increasing carbohydrates. The only dietary intervention studied thus far has been the effect of increased intake of complex carbohydrates. In a small study, women who ate carbohydrate-rich, protein-poor meals during the second half of their cycles had less depression, tension, anger, confusion, sadness, and fatigue.[8] Perhaps the cravings you have during the premenstrual period are for those things that your body knows will make it feel better (for more on healthy diets see chapter 5).

Some of these suggestions seem to make sense. Decreasing salt may help with fluid-retention symptoms. Caffeine may make you feel more anxious and irritable, so cutting back may help these symptoms. Alcohol can also affect your moods. However, none of these dietary changes has been proven as effective. But you can always try these dietary changes and see if they make a difference in you. After all, they are not harmful and if they help reduce your symptoms, you may need no further treatment.

Stress Reduction Approaches

Use of relaxation techniques have been studied and seem to help with PMS symptoms.[9] Stress appears to worsen PMS symptoms. Reduction of this stress through relaxation methods may help not only stress in general, but also the increased tension and stress a woman may feel during the premenstrual period. Relaxation techniques are probably good for overall mental, emotional, and physical health and are advisable for everyone to learn.

Vitamin and Mineral Supplements

Before taking any supplements or medication, be sure to discuss it with your physician. As outlined in chapter 10, supplements, though natural, may have significant risks. Vitamins B6 and E as well as magnesium and calcium have been used for PMS with varying results. (See chapter 10 for more information on vitamins and magnesium.)

Calcium Carbonate

Calcium, which you should be taking for your bones, has also been shown to be helpful in reducing PMS symptoms. There is some evidence that suggests a disturbance in calcium regulation may be involved in PMS. Women in one large study who took 1,200 mg of calcium in the form of two TUMS-EX twice a day had about a 50 percent reduction in overall PMS symptoms.[10] Calcium appeared to help with both mood and physical symptoms. (See chapter 11 for more information about calcium.)

Hormonal Options

Natural Progesterone

Progesterone supplements have been a popular form of treatment for PMS. A popular theory was that PMS was caused by a progesterone deficiency and that treatment with progesterone would be beneficial. This theory was popularized by Katarina Dalton, a general practitioner from England, through her book *Premenstrual Syndrome and Progesterone Therapy.*[11]

The evidence she presented for the effectiveness of vaginal progesterone suppositories for PMS was essentially a large series of case studies. In other words, women who had PMS tried the progesterone suppositories and many of them had improved symptoms. There was no control group of women taking placebo to make sure the improvement seen wasn't due to the placebo response. And this is a problem because of the high placebo response that results from any treatment for PMS. Since that time a review of studies comparing progesterone, either as a vaginal suppository or taken orally, with placebo showed no overall significant improvement of PMS symptoms over placebo.[12] At this time, progesterone supplements do not appear to be effective in treating PMS. (For more information about progesterone please see chapter 9.)

Combination Birth Control Pills

Birth control pills containing both estrogen and progestins (synthetic compounds that act like progesterone) have been used for PMS. Few studies have actually looked at the effectiveness of this approach. One study showed reduction of physical symptoms but not mood symptoms in women taking birth control pills.[13]

Birth control pills also have a number of side effects including moodiness, depression, nausea, and breast tenderness, especially when first started (see chapter 7). There is also some evidence that birth control pills may worsen PMS in some women.[14]

Birth control pills may be an option if you have no risks to taking the pill and need an effective form of contraception. The pill may also be reasonable if most of your symptoms are physical.

Danazol

Danazol is a synthetic androgen ("male" hormone) that can suppress ovulation when given in high enough doses. Once ovulation is suppressed, the hormones don't cycle normally. Danazol has been shown to help PMS but because of the side effects many women stopped using it.[15] Side effects of danazol include weight gain, facial hair growth, acne, deepening of the voice, and a decrease in HDL (the good cholesterol). Because of these and other potential side effects danazol is infrequently used.

Gonadotropin-Releasing Hormone (GnRH) Agonists

The symptoms of PMS end after menopause. This is because the hormones are no longer cycling, but are at a constant low level. When GnRH agonists are given to women, they shut down the ovaries, causing a temporary menopausal state. The PMS symptoms then resolve themselves.

The only problem is you've now traded PMS symptoms for menopausal symptoms such as hot flashes and night sweats. Some estrogen and progesterone can be given back to help alleviate the menopausal symptoms and usually do not cause a recurrence of the PMS.

There are several obstacles to the use of GnRH agonists. First are the menopausal side effects. These can be alleviated by the use of hormones. Second is cost. GnRH agonists are expensive, potentially costing thousands of dollars for a year of treatment. Thirdly, it has not been studied for long-term use—that is, for over a year. This is because it is not necessarily good for your body to stay in a menopausal state for a long period of time before you would naturally go through menopause. However, if the PMS symptoms are severe enough and other treatment options have failed to help, this may be an option to consider. (For more information on GnRH agonists, see chapter 3.)

Other Prescription Medications

Serotonin Reuptake Inhibitors (SSRIs)

Serotonin reuptake inhibitors (SSRIs) are a class of antidepressants that are thought to work by improving serotonin activity in the brain. Serotonin is a neurotransmitter (a chemical that let nerves communicate with each other) that may be linked to PMS. This may explain why SSRIs are effective in treating PMS.

There are now a large number of studies showing the effectiveness of SSRIs on treating PMS. Fluoxetine (Prozac) and sertraline (Zoloft) have been studied the most, but studies also show paroxetine (Paxil), citalopram (Celexa), and venlafaxine (Effexor) to be effective.[16] SSRIs can be taken continuously but have also been shown to be equally or possibly more helpful when taken during the two weeks before a period.

Side effects include insomnia, sedation, nausea, diarrhea, headache, dizziness, anxiety, decreased libido, difficulty having orgasm, and strange dreams. Generally, the side effects from SSRIs are mild and resolve over time. The sexual problems and weight gain can become a problem if these medications are used over a long period of time.[17] Taking SSRIs intermittently, for the second half of the cycle, may help reduce some of these side effects.

Of all the treatment options tried to date for PMS, SSRIs have shown to improve symptoms the most with minimal side effects. Yet many women with even severe PMS symptoms are reluctant to take them. The biggest problem many women have with taking SSRIs is the stigma that they believe is attached to these medications. Some women feel that taking these medications means that they are "mentally unstable" or that they're not strong enough to handle the hormonal changes.

Think of it this way. If you had bad cramping for one week out of the month and someone offered you something that would help it with minimal side effects, would you consider it? We're not suggesting everyone with PMS needs medications. As for any other medical condition, medicines should be considered only if the symptoms are severe and nothing else has worked. Like cramping, the symptoms will eventually resolve when you finish going through menopause.

Nonsteroidal Anti-Inflammatory Drugs (NSAIDs)

*N*onsteroidal *a*nti-*in*flammatory *d*rugs or NSAIDs are a class of medications that include ibuprofen (the active ingredient in Motrin and Advil) and naproxen sodium (Aleve, Anaprox, Naprelan, Naprosyn). These medications help with pain and decrease inflammation. Two medications in this class, naproxen sodium (Aleve, Anaprox, Naprelan, Naprosyn) and mefenamic acid (Ponstel) have also been shown to help reduce PMS symptoms.

Women taking naproxen sodium 550 mg twice a day or mefenamic acid 500 mg three times a day had a significant reduction of physical symptoms (headache, fatigue, and other pain) and mood symptoms (tension, irritability, and mood swings) over placebo.[18] These medications were started about one week before the start of the period and continued through the first few days of bleeding. Other benefits of this therapy include decreased cramping and bleeding during the menstrual cycle.

NSAIDs are generally well tolerated and relatively inexpensive. They should be taken with food as they can irritate the stomach, potentially leading to ulcers. Care should be taken not to take too much of these medications. If one NSAID, for example naproxen sodium, is being taken, another such as ibuprofen should not be taken at the same time. Taking too much can potentially damage the kidneys.

Antianxiety Medications

Antianxiety medications such as alprazolam (Xanax) have been shown to be somewhat helpful with PMS symptoms, mainly those of mood (mood swings, irritability, anxiety, and depression) and mental function (insomnia, poor coordination, confusion, and fatigue). However, the response is limited.[19] Given the side effects of these medications (such as sedation and lightheadedness and the potential to develop a tolerance and dependence to them, potentially leading to addiction), this class of medications should generally be limited to short-term use.

Spironolactone

Spironolactone is a diuretic or "water pill." It helps you get rid of fluid from your body. Given that one of the premenstrual symptoms is fluid retention, diuretics have been used to alleviate this problem. Spironolactone is the only diuretic that has been shown to help with PMS symptoms.

Women taking spironolactone 100 mg per day during the second half of their cycle were found to have decreased irritability, depression, breast tenderness, swelling, and food cravings. Another study found improvement only with bloating.[20] There are potentially serious side effects with this medication; as with all medications, it should be taken only under the direction of your physician.

Herbal and Alternative Remedies

Many alternative and herbal therapies (such as evening primrose and chasteberry) have been used to treat PMS but well-done studies are lacking in the medical literature, which make it difficult to assess their effectiveness. This does not mean that they are not effective, we just don't have proof at this time. And just because the remedies may be natural does not necessarily make them safer. In fact, the reverse may be true. (For more information on natural remedies see chapter 10.)

Surgical Options

Removal of the Ovaries (Oopherectomy)

PMS ends after a woman goes through menopause. This makes sense because when a woman goes through menopause, hormone levels stay constant: there is no more cycling of the hormones to trigger PMS. GnRH agonists are one way to temporarily put a woman into the menopausal state. The other way is to induce menopause permanently by removing the ovaries.

Nonetheless, surgical removal of the ovaries should be considered only as a last resort measure for severe PMS.[21] The ovaries can be removed alone or as part of a hysterectomy. (See chapter 3 for the pros and cons of removing the ovaries.)

Before considering surgery, you have to make sure you actually have PMS. If you have another problem such as depression, it will not be helped by surgery. And you certainly don't want to have surgery if it isn't going to help. The best way to determine if surgery may help is to take GnRH agonists (which will medically induce menopause) for at least four to six months. If your PMS symptoms resolve, then this would be a good sign that removing the ovaries may help.

If you are in your late forties and will soon be going through menopause anyway, you may just want to wait, or seriously consider GnRH agonists or other medication to hold you until you go through menopause naturally. This would save you from having surgery.

If you are younger than forty, you may want to consider seriously whether the premature menopause and the long-term lack of estrogen and other hormones will be worth the benefit. You also have to be sure you don't want any more children. Once you have your ovaries removed, you can't go back. It's irreversible and permanent. Fortunately, most women have significant improvement of their symptoms through other less drastic measures and rarely would need to consider this option.

So What's a Woman to Do about PMS?

With all these options, what's a woman in perimenopause to do? If your symptoms are mild like those of most women, regular aerobic exercise, calcium supplements, and stress-reduction techniques are the ideal place to start because of their general health benefits. Exercise is good for your heart, bones, and mind; calcium is good for your bones; and relaxation techniques are good for your mind. Cutting down on simple sugars and salt is also healthy for you and should be considered.

If you have no improvement after two to three cycles or if your symptoms are more severe, what you try next depends on your personal views on the different options. You may want to discuss the following possibilities with your physician: vitamin B6, magnesium, and NSAIDs. They are reasonable options that have few minor side effects if taken in sensible amounts.

If the symptoms are causing significant problems with your relationships or with work and none of the simpler options have worked, it is probably time to discuss further therapies with your physician.

DEPRESSION

In 1906, Emil Kraeplin identified "involutional melancholia" as a distinct syndrome. He defined the disorder as a depression that started during the "involutional years" or midlife.[22] Since that time, the relationship of hormonal changes with depression has been the center of debate. Many people still associate perimenopause and menopause with depression.

There are several types of depression: major depression, dysthymia, and bipolar disorder. Major depression is manifested by a combination of symptoms that interfere with work, sleep, and the enjoyment of pleasurable activities. Dysthymia is a less severe form of depression that involves long-term chronic symptoms that are not disabling, but keep a person from feeling good. Bipolar disorder (also known as manic-depressive illness) is characterized by cycling mood changes from episodes of feeling manic (high) to depression (low).

Depressive disorders may run in families. People with low self-esteem, who are readily overwhelmed by stress, and consistently view themselves and the world with pessimism are prone to depression. Depression may also be sparked by a serious loss, difficult relationships, and/or stressful events, although many people can have depression without a triggering event. So it may be a combination of genetic, psychological, and environmental factors that contribute to the onset of a depressive disorder. Nonetheless, the role of the changing hormones during perimenopause and menopause with depression is still open to debate.

What Is Depression?

Depression is a serious illness that can affect the way you feel, think, and act in a negative way. People with depression have a variety of symptoms, with a deep feeling of sadness being the most common. The diagnosis of major depression is made if a person has five or more of the following symptoms, which must include one of the first two symptoms for at least two consecutive weeks:[23]

- Feelings of sadness
- Loss of interest or pleasure in usual activities
- Changes in appetite that result in weight losses or gains not related to dieting
- Insomnia or oversleeping
- Loss of energy or increased fatigue
- Restlessness or irritability
- Feelings of worthlessness or inappropriate guilt
- Difficulty thinking, concentrating, or making decisions
- Thoughts of death or suicide or attempts at suicide

The symptoms cannot be due to physical illnesses, alcohol, medications, or substance abuse.

One in four women will have depression at some point in their lives. Currently, the cause of depression is thought to be related to an imbalance of certain neurotransmitters (chemicals that let nerves communicate with each other) in the brain. There also seems to be a genetic component to depression as it can run in families.

Why Is Depression More Common during Perimenopause?

There are different theories on why depression may be more common at this time, though once again, this topic is still controversial. The first theory emphasizes the hormonal changes as the precipitating factor for depression. Changes in hormone levels can cause mood changes, the most common example being PMS. And though PMS may worsen during perimenopause due to dropping hormone levels, this may not necessarily lead to depression. The physical changes such as insomnia and hot flashes caused by the dropping hormone levels may also contribute to the changes in mood. Poor sleep and fatigue can affect anyone's moods.

Another theory contends that the depression develops because of negative life events that tend to occur at this age. Children leaving the home, declining health, elderly parents who are sick, and changes in relationships may cause significant stress. There are also changes in a woman's body that lead to a feeling of loss. In this society, youthful attractiveness is highly prized, especially in women. At this time in life, there is also a realization that many dreams may not come to pass. Perhaps it's a lost career or not having children or an imperfect relationship. Whatever it is, the loss of a dream can also be very troubling.

How Is Depression Treated?

Medications for Depression

A number of medications are available for the treatment of depression. Most commonly used now are the class called serotonin reuptake inhibitors (see above). Other antidepressant medications are also available, such as heterocyclic antidepressants (which include tricyclic antidepressants) and monoamine oxidase inhibitors.

The heterocyclic antidepressants include amitriptyline, desipramine, doxepin, impramine, and nortriptyline. They can cause blurry vision, constipation, dry mouth, lightheadedness, and urinary retention. These side effects generally resolve over a few weeks. Rarely, more serious side effects can occur.

Monoamine oxidase inhibitors are even less commonly used because of dietary restrictions. People on this medication should not eat foods containing the amino acid tyramine found in cheese, beans, coffee, and chocolate among other foods. The tyramine can interact with this antidepressant and cause a severe and life-threatening increase in blood pressure. Monoamine oxidase inhibitors can also interact with other medications.[24]

Estrogen and Depression

Whatever the cause, if the depression is causing significant problems, medications and counseling are available. The use of estrogen in the treatment of depression in perimenopausal and postmenopausal women is controversial. Estrogen has been shown to help improve moods and several studies have shown that it may help with depressive symptoms in perimenopausal women.[25] Estrogen may also improve responsiveness to traditional antidepressants in postmenopausal women.[26] However, estrogen poses certain risks and is not considered a primary treatment option for depression and should mainly be used as an adjunct to help with other significant symptoms (for more information on estrogen, see chapter 9).

St. John's Wort (*Hypericum perforatum*)

A number of studies have shown St. John's wort to be more effective than placebo in treating mild to moderate depression. However, like other herbal remedies, there are potential risks and side effects when taking it. (For more information about St. John's wort, please see chapter 10.)

Depression and PMS

Symptoms of depression may also worsen before your periods. Premenstrual syndrome can combine with depressive symptoms to magnify the symptoms of depression, making the symptoms worse before your periods. Generally, treatment of depression will also help the PMS. If antidepressants are prescribed, sometimes an increase in the medication during the week or two before menstruation can be used to help keep the PMS under control. Again, check with your health care professional before ever increasing your dosage.

Physical Activity and Depression

Regular physical activity is good for the brain and helps with moods. Women who participate in regular physical activity have better mental health and less depression.[27] Physical activity has a plethora of other health benefits that cannot be overlooked and should be a part of your overall health regimen.

Suicide

The most devastating complication of depression is suicide. If you have severe symptoms of depression, feeling like your life is not worth living any more, or you have thoughts about hurting or killing yourself, you need immediate help. Call your physician, a suicide hotline (such as 800-SUI-CIDE), or 911 now to get help.

Now you may feel "depressed" but not have a diagnosis of "depression." Even if you don't meet the criteria for depression but the symptoms are significantly impacting your quality of life, treatment options are available. See a counselor, psychotherapist, psychologist, or physician right away.

THE BOTTOM LINE

PMS, depression, and other mood changes may be something you face during perimenopause and menopause. Whether or not these problems are related to hormonal changes, the treatment is still the same. Regular physical activity, a healthy diet, and adequate sleep are key aspects that help improve your overall physical, mental, and emotional health. Stress reduction, maintaining close relationships with friends and family, and remaining involved in activities that are meaningful to you are also very important to your overall health. However, should you develop any signs of depression or significant problems with PMS, you should seek the help of health care professionals.

CHAPTER 5

PACKING ON THE POUNDS

W eight—it's just a simple number we see when we step on the scale, but it's also a series of digits that can cause dismay when they increase and generally relief when they don't change or decrease. Many women become fixated on this number and its fluctuations. Unfortunately, weight tends to increase with advancing age. Starting in their late thirties many women notice that the activity level and diet previously needed to maintain their weight is no longer adequate: "I'm eating the same and just as active, but I'm gaining weight."

Interestingly, we are one of the most overfed, undernourished people in the world. We eat too much of the bad stuff and not enough of the good. The abundance and availability of energy-dense foods makes it easier to consume more calories than we need. That, combined with our sedentary lifestyle, is a recipe for added weight.

A decrease in the level of our physical activity may have contributed significantly to the increase in our weight in this country. A major barrier to physical activity may be the age in which we live, where modern technology has significantly reduced the amount of energy needed to perform most activities of daily living. These advances have also created sedentary leisure activities that often dominate our free time, such as watching television, playing video games, and surfing the Web.

An expanding waistline doesn't just impact the way your clothes fit or how you view yourself. It can also have a major impact on your health. A number of health problems are related to being overweight such as heart disease, diabetes, arthritis, and even certain cancers.

THE SIZE OF THE PROBLEM

According to the Third National Health and Examination Survey (NHANES III), a survey that collects information about the health and diet of people in the United States, slightly over half of all women twenty and older are overweight or obese. Since 1960 to 1994, this percentage has increased from 38.7 percent to 50.7 percent, with the largest increase in the previous decade. Current National Health and Examination Survey data show this trend continuing.[1] With respect to age, there is an increase in overweight and obese women with advancing age.

Age	20–29	30–39	40–49	50–59	60–69	70–79	80+
Percent overweight and obese	33.1	47.0	52.7	64.4	64.0	57.9	50.1

What Exactly Is Meant by "Overweight" and "Obese"?

The definitions of the terms overweight and obese are somewhat arbitrary. NHANES defines overweight and obesity in terms of body mass index or BMI. BMI uses height and weight to come up with a number that provides a more accurate measure of total body fat compared to using weight alone. BMI is measured as kilograms per meter squared (kg/m^2) and is calculated by taking your weight in kilograms and dividing by your height in meters squared. Or you can calculate it by taking your weight in pounds, multiplying it by 703 and then dividing by your height in inches squared.

$$\frac{\text{(your weight in pounds)} \times 703}{\text{(your height in inches)} \times \text{(your height in inches)}} = \text{your body mass index}$$

For example, if you weigh 150 pounds and are 5 feet 3 inches (63 inches) tall, you would multiply 150 (your weight) by 703, which would equal 105,450 (the top number). Multiply 63 (your height in inches) by itself and you will get 3,969 (the bottom number). Then divide 105,450 by

3,969 and the answer is 26.6, which would be your BMI. You could also look at the chart below to calculate your BMI.

Using the NHANES definition, overweight is a BMI of 25 to 29.9 kg/m². Obesity is a BMI over 30 kg/m².

	BMI (kg/m²)
Underweight	<18.5
Normal weight	18.5–24.9
Overweight	25–29.9
Obesity	≥30

Body Mass Index (BMI)

Weight in pounds

Height in feet and inches	110	120	130	140	150	160	170	180	190	200	210	220	230	240	250
5′	21	23	25	27	29	31	33	35	37	39	41	43	45	47	49
5′2″	21	22	24	26	27	29	31	33	35	37	38	40	42	44	46
5′4″	19	21	22	24	26	28	29	31	33	34	36	38	40	41	43
5′6″	18	19	21	23	24	26	27	29	31	32	34	36	37	39	40
5′8″	17	18	20	21	23	24	26	27	29	30	32	34	35	37	38
5′10″	16	17	19	20	22	23	24	26	27	29	30	32	33	35	36
6′	15	16	18	19	20	22	23	24	26	27	28	30	31	33	34
6′2″	14	15	17	18	19	21	22	23	24	26	27	28	30	31	32

Underweight	Normal weight	Overweight	Obesity

Health Risks Associated with Increasing Weight

Above a BMI of 20 kg/m², there is an increase in a number of health problems as the BMI increases. Health problems associated with being overweight or obese include:[2]

- Heart disease
- Stroke
- Diabetes
- High blood pressure

- Gallstones
- High cholesterol and triglycerides (a type of fat found in the blood)
- Arthritis
- Sleep apnea and other respiratory problems
- Breast cancer
- Endometrial cancer
- Colon cancer
- Kidney cancer
- Gallbladder cancer
- Urinary incontinence
- Psychological problems such as depression
- Menstrual irregularities
- Unwanted hair growth
- Decreased life expectancy

How much does being overweight increase some of these risks?[3]

- Heart disease: the risk is lowest if the BMI is 22 or less. A BMI of 25 to 28.9 doubles the risk, and 29 and over triples the risk.
- Stroke: a BMI of greater than 27 increases the risk 75 percent while a BMI of greater than 32 increases the risk 137 percent compared to a woman having a BMI of less than 21.
- Diabetes: the risk of diabetes increases by 25 percent for each BMI point over 22.
- Breast cancer: a weight gain of over 20 pounds from age eighteen to menopause doubles the risk of breast cancer.
- Colon cancer: a BMI of over 29 doubles the risk of distal colon cancer over women with a BMI of less than 21.

There is a decrease in life expectancy among overweight and obese women. Forty-year-old *nonsmoking* overweight women live 3.3 years less than women of normal weight. Obese *nonsmoking* women lose 7.2 years. These decreases in life expectancy are similar to those seen with smoking.[4]

The proportion of all deaths from cancer attributable to overweight and obesity may be as high as 20 percent among women over fifty in this country. This may be due not only to the excess weight increasing the risk of having cancer, but also to decreased ability to diagnose the cancer and/or respond to treatment for the cancer.[5]

Interestingly enough, animal studies have shown that animals fed diets with 30 percent fewer calories than animals who ate what they wanted lived significantly healthier and longer lives.[6] How this helps is still unclear. Possibly the decrease in food intake exposes the body to fewer toxins and other harmful substances such as cholesterol. Though it is unlikely anyone would be willing to maintain a 30 percent reduction in calorie intake for the majority of their adult lives, perhaps a smaller reduction may also be beneficial if for no other reason than to help with weight control.

The increase in these medical problems is the main reason to avoid significant weight gain or to try to lose weight if considerably overweight. Even if you already have some of these problems, weight loss will help control and prevent them from worsening. You may even be able to reverse the course of some diseases such as diabetes and be able to get off medications if you lose enough weight. Reducing your weight by even 10 percent will significantly improve your health.[7]

Are You an Apple or a Pear?

Where the weight is gained also affects your physical well-being. All fat is not the same. Weight gain that is more localized around the waist (giving a person the shape of an apple) rather than the hips or thighs (the pear shape) is associated with more health problems.

Women with a waist circumference of greater than thirty-five inches have a higher risk of heart disease, diabetes, high blood pressure, and cholesterol problems over that based on the BMI alone.[8] The waist circumference is measured by using a tape measure around the waist at the level of the top of the pelvic bones on the sides (see figure 5.1). The tape measure should be level with the floor. Hold it snug, but don't pinch the skin, and measure at the end of a breath after you have exhaled.

Is Weight Gain Related to Menopause?

There is some controversy whether weight gain during the time around menopause is related to the changes in hormones or simply to aging. The average woman gains two to five pounds during the menopausal transition.[9] Women going through

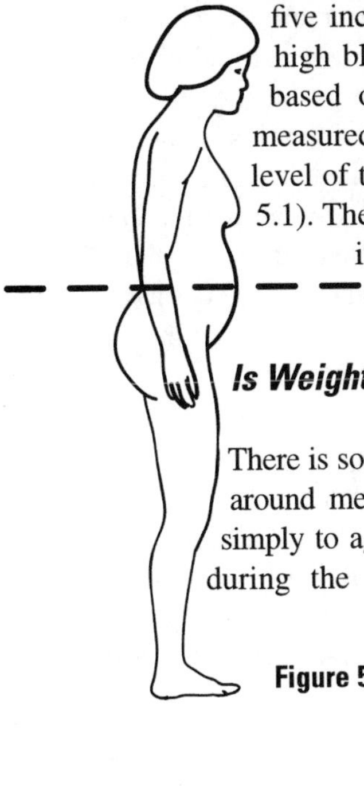

Figure 5.1. *Where to measure your waist circumference.*

menopause gain more body fat, especially in the waist; lose fat-free mass (such as muscle mass); and have a decrease in their resting metabolic rate.[10]

Regardless of whether the weight changes are related to menopause or just to aging, there are a number of factors that contribute to weight gain. With less muscle, there is less active tissue to burn calories, which contributes to the drop in metabolism. And the loss of muscle and increase in fat may be partially related to a decline in physical activity that is common during perimenopause and menopause.[11] In the past, the use of hormones was blamed for weight gain. However, studies have shown that hormone therapy does not increase the amount of weight gained after menopause. What they show is that all women, regardless of hormone use, tend to gain weight as they go through menopause.[12]

What about Genetic Factors?

Overweight people tend to come from families that are overweight. How much of it is genetic versus environmental—including the types of activities and diet encouraged—in a given family? The genetic contribution to BMI may be significant, but unfortunately it does little to help us address this problem.

Even if it were to be determined that there was a large genetic influence on weight, the approach and treatment would still be the same because those genetic factors cannot be changed. So if you were born into a heavy family, don't throw your hands up and decide that there's nothing you can do about it. Though you may be predisposed to gain more weight, you are still in control. You may have to work harder to lose and maintain your weight, but it can be done and you are the only one who can do it.

Remember, there has been a major jump in weight in this country over the past ten or twenty years. Our genes have not changed significantly over this time. We had the same genes a hundred years ago, but the number of overweight people were far fewer back then. Granted, life was much different back then, but it goes to show that having certain genes does not necessarily determine your fate concerning weight. The major culprit is an environment that promotes behaviors that cause weight gain.

SO WHAT'S CAUSING THE WEIGHT GAIN?

At the most basic level, if more calories are taken in than used, the excess calories are stored in the body as fat. Fat is your body's way of storing energy for later use when there may be less food available. For most of human history, that was an ideal way to save the extra calories because food was often scarce and the stored fat helped keep a person going until more food could be found. But now, for most people in this country, food is always so readily available that we rarely have to call on our fat stores to keep us going. The environment that we live in is dramatically different than in the past and is contributing to our current weight problem.

Decreased Physical Activity

The industrial revolution has changed the way we live, with machines doing much of our work so less "manpower" is needed. Our lives have become more sedentary. We have cars, buses, and trains to transport us, making it unnecessary to walk or ride a bicycle. We have machines to wash and dry our clothes, heaters for our homes so we don't have to chop and carry wood, and indoor plumbing so we don't have to pump and carry water.

For most of us, our jobs do not require much physical labor. We take elevators instead of stairs. We park our cars as close to the entrance as possible and drive from one side of a shopping center to the other to avoid walking. Sedentary leisure activities such as television, computers, and spectator events dominate our free time. And because we have packed our schedules with so many activities, we have little time or energy to exercise. So we now use fewer calories on our activities of daily living.

"Exercise" was unnecessary in the past because so much energy was expended during the course of a normal day. The need for exercise is a modern problem as our lives have become more sedentary. There is a cost to exercise, whether it is financial, such as joining a health club, or the loss of leisure time. But it is worth it.

Increased Calorie Intake

We have a dazzling array of tasty, inexpensive, convenient, and energy-dense foods (foods that are packed with calories) nearly everywhere we turn. Our hectic schedules make it more difficult to prepare healthy meals, so we eat more of these energy-dense foods. Making this problem worse is the trend toward larger portions. Fast food restaurants have led this trend by offering "super size" portions. Between 1977 and 1996, portion sizes increased for foods both inside and outside of the home.[13] The convenience and availability of energy-dense foods in larger servings have made it easier for us to consume more calories.

These modern changes have improved our lives dramatically, but have also made it much easier to gain weight. So in this land of abundance and leisure, our bodies have not adjusted to these changes and continue to hoard the calories and store them as fat, waiting for the rainy day when there is no more food. But the food keeps coming and the fat keeps accumulating. In their zeal to protect us, our bodies now turn on us.

HOW DO YOU LOSE THE WEIGHT?

The only way to lose weight is to use more calories than you eat. Sounds simple enough: eat less, be more active. Here again, there are many forces against you—some obvious, some not.

As you get older, your metabolic rate slows down.[14] Even if you eat the same and maintain your activity level, your weight will increase because you're burning fewer calories. So you have to decrease your intake or increase activity or both to maintain your weight. And if you want to lose weight, you have to work significantly harder than when you were younger.

You want to also try to balance your energy intake throughout the day. Unfortunately, because of work and family schedules, the biggest meal of the day is dinner, which is soon followed by sleep, which uses the least amount of energy. That means that much of those dinner calories becomes stored as fat. Ideally, if you keep the caloric intake the same, you would eat more at breakfast and lunch so that those calories are used for your daily activities.

Another problem is that once the fat accumulates, our bodies work to keep it. In the past, this probably was a way to protect against starvation, but now it makes it difficult to lose weight. As you eat less and lose weight, your body's metabolism slows and these changes may persist for months or years, making it more difficult to maintain the weight loss.[15] Basically, as you lose weight, your body thinks that there's a famine and works to use as little energy as possible.

But despite these obstacles, you can still overcome and triumph. It's just more difficult. So what can you do?

Watch What You Eat

What are you supposed to eat in order to lose weight? Do you cut out the fat and increase the carbohydrates? Or do you hold the carbs and eat all the protein and fat you want? With all the diets out there, it's confusing to figure out what's the best way to maintain or lose your weight. Most of the diet plans have their supporters and detractors. So what's right?

Most people can lose weight using any number of diets. The main problem is keeping off what you lose. A better way is to change the way you look at eating and food. You may be thinking that you'll diet, and once the weight is off, you get to go back to your old habits. Instead, you need to change the way you eat—permanently.

So rather than going on a radical diet with major changes in what you eat, think about modifying what you are already eating. This way, you'll be more likely to continue this way of eating for the long term.

Drinks: A Quick Way to Take in Calories

One major source of empty calories is drinks. Fruit juices and soft drinks are the biggest culprits. A twelve-ounce can of cola contains about 140 calories; 3,500 calories equal one pound of weight.[16] If you cut out one can of cola a day and you don't change anything else, you could lose about fourteen pounds in one year.

A twelve-ounce glass of orange juice contains 180 calories. Many people feel that juices are healthy and good for them, providing vitamins, potassium, and other nutrients. They are healthier for you than colas, but it is much better for you to eat the fruit rather than drink the juice because the fruit will help fill you up and provide fiber and other nutrients that are missing from the juice. And though juice is completely natural and may not have any added sugar, fruit juices still have a high content of fructose, which is a simple sugar not unlike refined sugar. So if you cut out one glass of orange juice a day, you could lose about eighteen pounds in one year.

Alcohol is another source of calories that you can reduce or eliminate. A twelve-ounce can of beer has 140 calories, while four ounces of wine has about 80. Mixed drinks such as margaritas and pina coladas can have plenty of calories because of the sugary mixtures added to the alcohol. Some people drink alcohol because of possible health benefits—but alcohol may also cause significant problems (see chapter 13).

Try to cut out any drinks that have a significant number of calories. Drinks are an easy way to take in a lot of calories that don't satisfy your hunger. Substitute diet drinks, flavored noncaloric sparkling water, or better yet, water for sodas, fruit juices, sweet tea, and sweetened drinks. If you drink those specialty coffee drinks, many of them are packed with calories. Go back to regular coffee and use skim or low-fat milk instead of cream. Even if you use sugar it will have far fewer calories than those specialty coffees.

Alter Your Eating Habits

If you eat fast food regularly for lunch at work or home, start making your own lunch. Make a sandwich with whole wheat bread. Look at the ingredients on the label. Some breads look like wheat but are still made with enriched wheat flour. You want bread made of whole wheat flour (lower glycemic index and more fiber; see below). Use turkey breast and if you must have cheese, use low-fat cheese. Hold the mayonnaise. That's a large source of fat and calories. Use mustard instead. To keep yur sandwich from getting soggy, pack lettuce or tomatoes in a separate plastic bag and add them to your sandwich before you eat it. Eat a piece of fruit. This will be much healthier, providing you with a wider variety of nutrients with significantly fewer calories than the fast-food lunch.

Try to change your snack foods. Instead of reaching for chips, cookies, or ice cream, snack on fresh fruits or veggies. If fruit doesn't quite hit your sweet spot, sweetened or unsweetened cold cereal isn't quite as healthy, but is another alternative that generally has fewer calories and less fat than the other snack foods.

Go from whole milk (150 calories per eight-ounce glass) to skim milk (90 calories). Hold the butter (100 calories per tablespoon) on your baked potato, bread, or other foods. Substitute reduced-fat Italian dressing (only 30 calories for two tablespoons) for regular Italian salad dressing (136 calories).

When you go out to eat, don't feel you have to finish the meal. Many restaurants are now serving larger portions. You can either split an entrée or you can always take a doggy bag home. Or you can order an appetizer as your main meal. Ask for the salad dressing on the side and use it sparingly. Most of the calories in salads are in the salad dressing. Don't be fooled into thinking that salads are better, because many are packed with calories from the dressing, cheese, croutons, and bacon bits.

Fat versus Carbohydrates: Which One Should You Cut?

In the past, the emphasis was on cutting out fat in the diet. The thought was that fat was bad for the heart and fat has more calories than protein and carbohydrates.

- one gram of fat = 9 calories
- one gram of carbohydrate = 4 calories
- one gram of protein = 4 calories

So each gram of fat has over twice the calories of each gram of protein or carbohydrate. Fat packs more energy ounce for ounce than protein or carbohydrates. That makes it easier to eat more calories in fat than protein or carbohydrates.

This push to lower fat intake led to low-fat foods and the illusion that cutting fat would lead to healthier bodies. The food industry responded by producing low-fat and no-fat foods that became very popular as people purchased them, believing that these foods were healthier. However, in terms of weight control, these low-fat alternatives did not pave the road to weight loss. This was because many of the low-fat alternatives had essentially the same number of calories as the original food. Sugar was added to these foods to make them more palatable. So people were eating the same number of calories, just in a different form.

However, fat may also help satisfy your hunger better so that you eat less. There are different types of fat and some are better for you than others. The goal, then, is to see what are the differences between the different fats to try and understand which ones you will want to eat. But remember, the different types of fats still have the same number of calories.

1. Saturated fats

- Solid at room temperature
- Include animal fats such as butter, lard, red meat, poultry skin, cheese, whole milk, ice cream, cream, and certain vegetable oils (coconut, palm, and palm kernel oils)
- Increases LDL (the bad cholesterol), and the risk of heart disease and strokes

2. Monounsaturated fats

- Liquid at room temperature but start to solidify in the refrigerator
- Includes plant oils such as olive, canola, and peanut oils and avocados
- May help lower cholesterol levels when used in place of saturated fats

3. Polyunsaturated fats

- Liquid at room temperature and in the refrigerator
- Includes plant oils such as safflower, sesame, soy, corn, and sunflower-seed oils, nuts, and seeds
- May help lower cholesterol levels when used in place of saturated fats

4. Transfatty acids

- Transfatty acids are unsaturated fats that have undergone a chemical change during food processing, making them more saturated
- Found in french fries, donuts, and other commercial fried foods as well as cookies, crackers, margarine, and vegetable shortenings
- Transfatty acids raise LDL (the bad cholesterol) and triglycerides, lower HDL (the good cholesterol), and increase the risk of diabetes and heart disease[17]
- Look at the ingredients—hydrogenated or partially hydrogenated vegetable oils are an indication of transfatty acids in foods

Overall, saturated fat and transfatty acids are the bad players. They tend to increase the risk of heart disease, diabetes, and stroke and should be avoided.[18] They may also affect the risk of other medical problems such as Alzheimer's disease. In one study, people who ate the most saturated fats and transfatty acids had more than double the risk of Alzheimer's disease than those who ate the least.[19]

In summary, the possible risks of saturated fats and transfatty acids are:

- Raised LDL (the "bad" cholesterol)
- Raised triglycerides
- Lowered HDL (the "good" cholesterol)
- Increased risk of heart disease
- Increased risk of strokes
- Increased risk of diabetes
- Increased likelihood of Alzheimer's disease

What about the low carbohydrate diets that have become so popular? They do seem to work. So are carbohydrates the bad stuff that should be avoided while fat is okay?

The answer is probably more complicated than a fat-versus-carbohydrate issue. The problem is that many of the recommendations in the past lumped all types of fats and all types of carbohydrates together. It appears that all fats and all carbohydrates are not the same when it comes to the way your body processes them and their effects.

Carbohydrates: More Than Meets the Eye

There are different types of carbohydrates. You've probably heard of simple and complex carbohydrates. Simple carbohydrates are simple sugars such as sucrose (table sugar) and fructose (fruit sugar) that are composed of small sugar molecules. Complex carbohydrates are composed of long strands of simple sugars. Examples of complex carbohydrates include starches and cellulose (fiber). The thought was that complex carbohydrates were better for you because they took longer to break down and were absorbed over a longer period of time.

The Glycemic Index

However, carbohydrates have more recently been studied to see how the body reacts to them when they are eaten. The recently coined term "glycemic index" indicates how quickly a carbohydrate increases the blood sugar level in the body. The higher the number, the more sugar and insulin levels rise.

High–glycemic index foods are rapidly absorbed by the body, leading to a quick rise in blood sugar levels. The rapid rise of sugar causes your body to release lots of insulin to bring the sugar levels back to a normal range. However, your body may release so much insulin that it causes a sharp drop in sugar levels to levels lower than normal. This causes hypoglycemia. Hypoglycemia is a condition in which the blood sugar levels are low and can cause headache, dizziness, shakiness, weakness, and irritability. Hypoglycemia leads to feelings of hunger, making you want to eat again, restarting this cycle.

Foods such as white bread, potatoes, pasta, and white rice have a high glycemic index. So some complex carbohydrates such as starch (found in potatoes) may not be as good for you as previously thought. High–glycemic index meals may promote overeating and may raise LDL (the "bad" cholesterol) and triglyceride (another kind of fat in the blood) levels. Long-term diets high in these foods may increase the risk of significant weight gain, diabetes, and heart disease.[20]

Eating low glycemic foods such as fruits and vegetables (containing lots of water), whole grains, and lean meats seems to curb hunger better than high glycemic foods. These foods also are less energy dense. Eating bulky foods such as fresh fruits and vegetables helps you feel full quicker so that you tend to eat less and still be satisfied.

Protein helps slow down absorption of food, reducing the glycemic index of a meal. By adding protein such as lean meats and soy foods to meals and snacks, you may help blood sugar levels rise more slowly so that you don't have the problems seen with high–glycemic index meals.

Change Your Diet to Fit Your Taste

So what to do? People do the best when they find a diet that works for their individual taste. No one diet plan will work for everyone. So try to modify your existing diet by eating foods high in fiber (such as whole grain foods) and relatively unprocessed carbohydrates (such as fresh fruits and vegetables), which are more filling. Cut back on sweet drinks and other simple carbohydrates. Decrease the amounts of saturated fats and transfatty acids, which have negative health consequences, and replace them with mono-unsaturated and polyunsaturated fats. But remember that all fats are more calorie dense than carbohydrates and protein so you want to limit them. Add protein to your meals and snacks.

Overall, you want to reduce your calorie intake. Only by decreasing your calorie intake, regardless of the source, will you be able to lose weight. But you can do it in a way that your hunger and taste buds are satisfied.

For a Healthier Diet

Increase	Decrease
Fruits and vegetables	High glycemic foods
Fiber	Saturated fats
Monounsaturated fats	Transfatty acids
Polyunsaturated fats	
Omega-3 fatty acids	
Lean proteins	

WHAT ABOUT EXERCISE?

Exercise is great for your health, but how effective is it to help with weight loss or weight maintenance? What you eat and drink provides calories to your body. Your body then uses those calories to carry out all your activities. By exercising or increasing your overall level of activity, you burn more calories. And that's the other side of the energy coin.

In general, however, more weight can be lost through diet than exercise. This makes sense because by cutting out one cola a day, you cut out about 140 calories coming into your body. You would have to walk about two miles to burn the same number of calories. To lose a pound a week by exercising alone, you would have to burn an extra 500 calories a day, the equivalent of walking about six miles a day. So in the overall energy equation of calories consumed and calories used, it's easier to cut than to burn the same number of calories.

> *To lose one pound of weight, you have to burn 3,500 more calories than you take in. To lose a pound a week by* exercising alone, *you would have to burn an extra 500 calories a day, the equivalent of walking about* six miles a day, every day.

That doesn't mean exercise doesn't have a role in weight loss and maintenance. The combination of diet and exercise is the most effective way to lose weight and keep it off. Exercise seems to be especially important in maintaining your weight. Exercise helps build muscles, which helps you burn more calories even at rest. Studies show that most people need to exercise to maintain their lower weight.[21]

How Much Exercise Is Needed to Lose Weight?

The amount of exercise needed to help lose weight is still unclear.[22] The public health recommendation of thirty minutes of physical activity of moderate intensity on most days of the week is based on the effect of exercise on heart disease and diabetes. This level of activity alone is probably not enough to produce weight loss or maintain it.

One study showed that women who were on a diet and exercised over 280 minutes a week (average of forty minutes every day) lost twice the weight and maintained that weight loss over women who dieted and exercised less.[23] That's significantly more exercise than most people do when trying to lose or maintain weight.

Before you give up and think that you can't exercise that much, remember that any increase in activity or exercise is better than none. Don't be discouraged if an exercise program doesn't seem to be decreasing your weight. Exercise still makes you healthier: it's good for your bones, heart, and mind.

Aerobic exercise seems to help more with weight loss than weight or resistance training (exercise where you strengthen muscles by pushing or pulling against something that resists you). However, weight and resistance training helps improve strength and build muscles; as we already mentioned, this in turn helps you burn more calories even at rest. Resistance training is also good for your bones, helps prevent falls, and is good for other aspects of daily life.

One thing to watch out for is the false belief that if you exercise, you can then splurge on your diet. As you can see in the table below, it takes quite a bit of effort to burn off extra calories.

Activity (from easiest to most strenuous)	Minutes to burn about 150 calories	Foods	Amount that contains about 150 calories
Washing windows or floors	45 to 60	Broccoli	3 cups
Playing volleyball	45	Apple	2 small
Gardening	30 to 45	Banana	1 and a half
Walking 20 min/mile	35	Wheat bread	2 slices
Bicycling 10 mph	30	Bagel	¾ of a bagel
Dancing fast	30	Cola	One can
Walking 15 min/mile	30	Hamburger regular	Half a burger
Water aerobics	30	Chocolate chip cookie	3 cookies
Aerobics, low impact	25	Cheesecake	Half of a slice
Swimming laps	20	Vanilla ice cream	Half cup
Jumping rope	15	Glazed doughnut	⅔ of a doughnut
Running 10 min/mile	15	Starbucks caffe Latte	8 ounces
Stairwalking	15	Milk chocolate candy	1 ounce

When you start an exercise program, start slowly and gradually increase the duration and intensity of the activity. Doing too much at once may make you feel like you're doing a lot, but you're more likely to quit when your body protests too much. If you feel you don't have the time, do a little here and a little there. Walk during your breaks. Take the stairs. Park farther away. Every little bit helps.

DIETARY SUPPLEMENTS

"Lose weight fast! No dieting, no exercise. Just take this pill and the pounds will just melt away." If it were only as easy as taking a pill to lose weight. There are medications as well as over-the-counter dietary supplements used to help with weight loss. Surgery is another option for people with severe weight problems. (Surgery and prescription medications are beyond the scope of this book and are topics that should be discussed with your physician.)

Over-the-counter dietary supplements are readily available to anyone. It's tempting to use one of these remedies to help with weight loss. "I'll use it only for a short time until I get the weight off," you say to yourself. Supplements containing ephedra (also known as ma huang) and caffeine products are widely used to help with weight reduction. They have been found to help modestly with short-term weight loss, but are also associated with adverse affects including high blood pressure, palpitations, stroke, seizures, and even death.[24]

Other weight loss products have also been found to have adverse side effects. LipoKinetix, which is sold as a dietary supplement for weight loss and contains phenylpropanolamine, caffeine, yohimbine, diiodothyronine, and sodium usniate has been associated with liver failure.[25]

Perhaps some of these problems occur in people who have underlying health problems that predispose them to having a reaction to these supplements. Unfortunately, dietary supplements are not well regulated and very few studies have been done to prove their efficacy or safety. So the best thing to do is avoid these dietary supplements and control your weight the old-fashioned (and harder) way.

Some tips to lose weight:

- Make changes that will work for you. Think of ways to permanently cut back on calories that fit your lifestyle and preferences.
- Eat smaller portions until you are satisfied, not stuffed.
- Cut back or eliminate sweetened drinks, including sodas and fruit drinks.

- Try to reduce the amount of high glycemic foods such as white bread, white rice, processed foods, sugar, and potatoes.
- Increase your intake of high fiber foods such as whole wheat bread, brown rice, and oatmeal.
- Increase fresh vegetables and fruits.
- Reduce the amount of saturated fats and transfatty acids and replace them with monounsaturated and polyunsaturated fats such as olive oil, avocados, nuts, and seeds.
- Eat lean proteins such as fish, chicken (without the skin), lean beef, and low- or no-fat dairy products with each meal.
- Increase your activity level. Take the stairs. Park farther away. Walk during breaks. Start an enjoyable hobby such as gardening or bird watching. Pick up a sport such as golf or tennis or just start walking regularly.
- If you are really motivated, start a more intensive aerobic and/or weight or resistance training program.

THE BOTTOM LINE

The best way to approach weight is to figure out what will work for you. Everyone is different and what works for one person may not work for another. You know your food likes and dislikes and what types of activities you enjoy. At this stage of your life, what you have to do is learn to look at food and activity in a different way and to make lifelong changes to maintain your weight and health.

To lose the weight, you have to modify your eating pattern so that you eat fewer calories than you burn. Start walking every day, even if it's only for five minutes. As you get in these new routines, you can gradually change more things and increase your activity level. Granted, the weight loss may be relatively slow, but if you maintain these changes, the weight will stay off and your overall health will improve. Extra weight gain at this time of life is not inevitable. Yes, it is harder to control your weight now than when you were younger. But you have a choice. You and only you can do it.

CHAPTER 6

NOT IN THE MOOD

I tell my husband, "You can do whatever you want. Just don't wake me up."

—Loretta Loughman

*I*f you have a satisfying sex life and your relationship with your significant other is going well, then that's wonderful and you can skip this chapter. If, on the other hand, you have noticed changes in your sexual functioning and a decline in your sex drive, you are not alone. Many women notice a change in their libido at this stage in their life. Some share their stories with their friends. Others approach their physicians with their questions. But most stay silent.

Changes that may occur during perimenopause and afterward that may affect your sex drive include:

- Loss of desire
- Decreased lubrication
- Decreased genital sensation
- Difficulty achieving orgasm
- Painful intercourse
- Issues regarding your partner

Changes in sex drive can become noticeable during perimenopause. A drop in libido usually causes the most problems. Hormones may possibly play a role in this, but other factors also need to be considered, such as relationship issues, fatigue, situational factors, medical problems, and medications. These changes are not uncommon and only recently have been discussed more openly. We will explore the causes and strategies that may be helpful in approaching this topic.

"NOT TONIGHT HONEY"

Sex. It's in the movies, on television, in music, on billboards, everywhere. You may feel everyone is doing it more often and enjoying it more than you, especially as your relationship matures from the initial hot and heavy romantic love into . . . what? This is a time in many women's lives when their relationship with their significant other has reached a plateau. According to some women's magazines, women reach their sexual peak in their midthirties. However, some women may try to figure out what is meant by peak because sex may seem at times to be more of a chore or duty than something to be desired.

Sex for Men and Women Is Different

Sex for men and women is different (surprise!). The book that said that men were from Mars and women were from Venus got it right.[1] Men, in general, can compartmentalize sex and separate it from other aspects of their lives. They can get fired at work, get bitten by a dog, get in a fight with you at dinner, but when they get into bed for the night, they look over and say, "Hey, let's have sex." Sex is not only just a physical desire but also a major way for a man to feel connected and close to his partner.

For a woman, physical intimacy is generally an extension of emotional intimacy. Most women in a relationship need to feel emotionally close to their partner before they want to be physically close. Unfortunately, for many women there are so many demands on their time through the years: raising children, helping with homework, carting them to extracurricular activities, taking care of the house, assisting aging parents, and on and on—as well as working to maintain their relationship with their significant other.

Figure 6.1

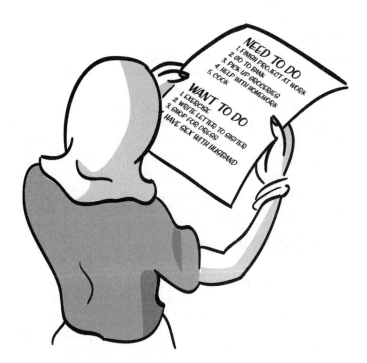

Changing Priorities

Unfortunately, with all the time demands, the significant other sometimes becomes a lower priority, especially in a long-standing relationship. So by the time the modern woman in her late thirties or older finally gets to bed, she wants at most to catch up with her partner before crashing to sleep in exhaustion. She may want to cuddle, but is afraid to, because that may lead her partner to think she wants more when she really doesn't.

Meanwhile, the male half of the partnership doesn't understand what's happening. In the past getting into bed was often followed by sex. Now, if his advances are rebuffed, he likely takes it personally. "You don't love me anymore." So he may sulk and pout. For a man, one of the ways he shows his affection and love for someone is through physical intimacy. He's generally not wired to show it in other ways. So when you reject his advances, he's likely to take it personally, no matter how much you tell him otherwise.

But you may see his sulkiness as his being demanding and selfish. "Can't he see how exhausted I am and just leave me alone?" When you were first together, even if you both had a busy day at work, you had the evening to connect and become emotionally closer so that by the time you got to bed, you were more likely to be physically intimate. Now, you are exhausted and tired of having bosses, coworkers, and children of whatever age asking you for this or that, draining your energy, and yet here is someone else who wants something from you. Many women spend their lives as givers and sometimes you just run out of gifts and want some time alone.

So there you are in bed, exhausted, your significant other sulking and upset at being rebuffed yet again, wondering if there is something wrong with you. It wasn't always this way. Overall, your relationship is good. When you do have sex, it's actually still pleasurable. In fact, right after you've been physically intimate, you may wonder why you've put it off for so long. "So what is wrong with me? Something must be wrong for me to feel this way." And it doesn't help that your partner is echoing those same thoughts. Is there really something wrong, is it an inevitable part of aging, or are there other reasons for this change?

The Evolution of Sex

From an evolutionary standpoint, it makes sense that your sex drive would decrease over time, especially after you have had children. Imagine back in the cave man days having countless children. It would have been difficult to protect, feed, and clothe them until they were old enough to fend for themselves. So perhaps there was a biologic incentive to decrease a woman's sex drive after having a few children.

Also, as you approach menopause, your fertility decreases; after menopause, you can no longer become pregnant. So sex after menopause is no longer a biologic necessity from a reproductive standpoint. Since sex no longer has a reproductive function for a woman, perhaps this is another evolutionary reason for the diminishing sex drive at this point in time. Men, on the other hand, can continue to reproduce and father children into their seventies and beyond, though they, too, slow down.

Does aging doom a woman to a life of sexual apathy? Are women programmed not to want to have sex after menopause when procreation is no longer possible? Well, sex is a lot more complicated than just hormones, organs, and technique. A survey of 2,001 Australian women aged forty-five to fifty-five showed that 31 percent had a decrease in sexual interest when going through natural menopause. However, 62 percent of the women showed no change in interest, and 7 percent actually had an increase in interest.[2] So the good news is that the majority of women do not seem to have a decline in their sexual interest during perimenopause.

However, women have different baseline levels of sexual desire and functioning, so there could be a change even before perimenopause. What are some of the factors that contribute to changing sexuality in women at this time?

DECREASING SEX DRIVE

Many women first notice a decrease in their sex drive in their mid to late thirties, usually after they have had a child or two or three. A number of factors probably contribute to this change. First, you are much more busy keeping up with your children, which is stressful and exhausting. Factors that are critical to a relationship such as communication, power struggles, differences in sex drive, and quality time spent together may also have an impact on your sex drive. Changing hormone levels during perimenopause may also play a role in this part of your life.

Fatigue and Stress

Once you've had children, your life, as you may well know, undergoes a major transformation. Each child demands and deserves your time. Whether or not you work outside of the home, you are not immune to the needs of your progeny. If you stay at home and have younger children, they require much of your attention, unless they go to daycare or school. Older children may need less direct supervision, but create their own unique set of mental and physical stress.

If you work outside of the house, when you get home multiple chores await you, from food to housekeeping to children's issues. Regardless, by the end of the day when the children are finally asleep, you are so tired that the most you might want to do is veg out in front of the television before slipping into that nocturnal oblivion known as sleep. For those women without children, many have demanding jobs (as do women with children) that sap their energy as well.

Fatigue and stress do little to improve your libido. At this point in your life, you're in catch-up mode: you're always trying to catch up on things that need to be done, one of them being sleep.

Figure 6.2

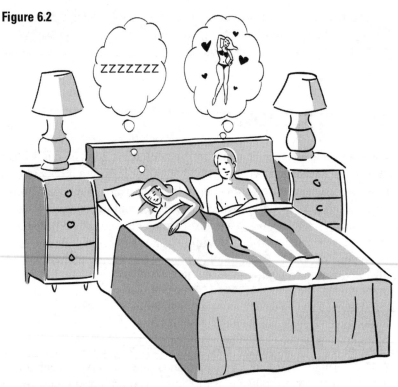

Too Many Things to Do

So many things to do, so little time. That is one of the curses of the modern family life. With the abundance available to us in this country, many of us feel compelled to partake in as many activities as we can cram into our already overloaded schedules, stressing us even further.

Unfortunately, something has to give. We can't do everything. As much as you have tried to be superwoman, you still have limitations. The first thing to suffer in our pursuit of the good life is quiet time and sleep. Constantly exhausted, you let your relationship with your significant other and sex slide lower on the priority scale. After all, sex takes energy.

When you reach menopause, your children may be older and less demanding in many ways, but now hot flashes, night sweats, and other factors conspire to rob you of sleep, which again results in fatigue. Stress from your adolescent or older children, stress from elderly parents, stress from your job, and other stressors affect your ability to rest. So once again, fatigue may interfere with your sex drive.

Interpersonal Issues

For most, sex, like dancing, is best done with a partner. And whenever you have two people together, even a well-matched couple, there can be conflict. Interpersonal issues, expectations about sex, and your partner's sexual problems are an important part of your sexual experience. After all, what's the biggest sex organ in your body? Your brain. It doesn't matter how lubricated and aroused your body may be—if your brain doesn't want sex, the rest doesn't matter.

Interpersonal issues are probably one of the biggest barriers to sex for a woman. Generally, women want to feel emotionally close to the person with whom they are sexually intimate. Not that this is true all of the time. Once in a while a woman may want something purely physical to explore her sexuality. However, if a woman is ambivalent about her relationship, it may likely negatively affect her sexual functioning and degree of satisfaction.

For many women, menopause is a time when they've reached a plateau in their relationships. The courtship has ended, romance may be lacking, and foreplay may be, "I'm ready, aren't you?" A multitude of priorities and stressors as well as a cooling of your relationship may lead to an increasing distance between you and your partner.

"Just Leave Me Alone"

You become tired of everyone always wanting, needing, reaching, grabbing, or asking for something from you, whether it's a boss, coworker, children, family, neighbor, or significant other. By late in the evening, you just want time to yourself with no demands on you. So you find yourself saying, "Sorry dear, not tonight," or some variation of it.

The fatigue and time needed to care for everything else eats into a couple's time. Quality one-on-one time with your significant other becomes very scarce or even nonexistent. As a result, communication breaks down and your relationship drifts further and further apart.

Power Struggles

Power struggles are another factor that may pull relationships apart. "I do all the work around the house. Why can't he help?" "She's always nagging me about things. Doesn't she know how tired I am?" "Why can't he see things my way?" "Why can't she see things my way?" Soon, each person is convinced that he or she is right and tries to convince the other to view the world through his or her perspective. So they both butt heads and argue, trying to prove their own point of view.

Relationships aren't about someone winning. If someone wins, someone loses—and in the long run, that will only hurt the relationship. Admitting that the other person has a point doesn't necessarily mean that you are wrong. Both partners need to appreciate each other's viewpoint. If not, what ends up happening is that names are called and feelings are hurt. The original reason for the argument may be long gone, but all that's left is a festering pain.

Relationships Take Work

Relationships are fragile. They are built on love and while the bonds of love can be amazingly strong, even they can falter and fail. Relationships are about respect and treating each other as equals. Relationships have to be nurtured. Though a relationship may bloom to life with new love, it is when your relationship begins to mature that it needs the most support. But for a relationship to grow and stay strong, you must pour your heart, love, and soul into it so that it continues to thrive, and is able to stand against almost anything.

Love can start a relationship, but only trust and respect can make it grow. Once you've laid the foundation of your relationship based on these basic precepts, it will grow. And this takes time. Time that you feel you may not have to spare. But you must make time if you want your relationship to succeed. Time, energy, and commitment, though, all are in woefully short supply.

Open lines of communication are the only way in which the relationship can continue to grow. Communication is the root through which the relationship gains the nutrients of love and respect. Cut off the lines of communication and you cut the root and the relationship will die.

Most problems in relationships are a result of poor communication. Poor communication leads to misunderstandings, a lack of awareness of each other's feelings, and a feeling of isolation—this is at the root of power struggles.

Time Together

Time. No matter where you live, no matter who you are, and no matter what you do, everyone has the same twenty-four hours in a day to do all the things they want to do. How do you squeeze in more time with your partner? Like anything else that's important in your life, you will have to schedule time together.

You should set up a "date" with your partner. When was the last time you and your partner spent time alone together? Not when the two of you were with your family, at a party with friends, or asleep in bed together, but time when the two of you actually were together and could talk without interruption? If you're like many of us, it's been awhile. And if so, it's time to set up a date. Or better yet, set up a regular schedule for dates, ideally, at least twice a month.

Before you think of all the reasons why you can't do it, ask yourself, Is my relationship with my partner important? If it's not important, it may already be too late. And if it is important, then this is something you have to do if you want your relationship to survive and thrive. Get a baby sitter, a trusted relative, or swap nights with a friend. If you have trouble leaving your children, go out after they go to sleep. Be creative. If you put your mind to it, you will find a way to escape with your partner.

It doesn't have to be expensive. And don't spend the whole time at a movie. You want time when you can talk and interact. Go out to eat. It needn't be a fancy restaurant. Share dessert or a cup of coffee. Don't forget, having two parents who love each other means a lot to your children.

If you absolutely can't get away, then schedule time when the two of you can sit outside and talk without being disturbed. Tell your children that you need time alone to talk. Telling each other what needs to be done while you pass in the hallway doesn't count. Even if you do have date nights, setting a time when you can spend time talking on a regular basis during the week is also very helpful for making your relationship stronger. If you set aside time during the week to take care of your family business, this will allow your date to be more free flowing and romantic.

Communicating

Communication is the key to understanding each other's needs. Most men are trainable. You could try to preface any discussion with, "I just want you to listen. I don't want you to try to solve the problem," or "I want you to know how I'm feeling. Don't say anything and just listen." The first couple of times, he may try to say something and you may have to remind him to just listen. But after a while, he may actually get it and understand what you want.

And if you want feedback, by all means, let him know, or he may stay in the "I'm supposed to be just listening and not talking" mode. Most men want to please their better half. It's just that they don't know what's expected of them many times and need it spelled out in black and white. Once they know the rules, they tend to respond much better.

And for those of you who feel that your partner should be more attuned to your feelings and know how to react, it will help both of you if you let him know more directly. If you voice your desire to share more of the family chores and tell him that this will free you up to have more time to be with him, he may well help more, which will provide more quality time for the two of you.

Many women feel disappointed or get frustrated when their partner doesn't seem to be attuned to things as she thinks he should be. But men are wired differently. They are much more concrete and need help in understanding these more intangible things. And only you can really help your partner to see this. Men are not mind readers. By the same token, you need to listen to your husband's thoughts without interruption and try to see his viewpoint.

DIFFERENCES IN SEX DRIVE

The approach to sexual problems in men and women is different. Men usually want to have sex. If they have a sexual problem, it is usually physical, the main one having or maintaining an erection. For women, the biggest problem is mental: wanting to have sex. That's why Viagra has worked so well for men; their sex drive was still there, they just couldn't do anything about it. Once Viagra helped them have an erection, they were ready to go.

Nonetheless, your partner may have medical problems or be on medications that may affect his ability to have an erection. If he can't have an erection, he may withdraw from you sexually and rebuff your advances. Or he may be under significant stress which can mentally affect his desire or performance.

Many women in relationships experience the opposite problem. Their partner wants to have sex more frequently than they do. This can lead to resentment on both sides: the man feels repeatedly rejected while the woman feels constantly pressured. Part of the problem can be a difference of opinion of how much sex is desirable. If there is a great mismatch in libido—say, for example, that the man would like to have sex every day but the woman would be happy with sex once a month or vice versa—this could lead to problems.

It's also a matter of expectations. Though some men would like to have sex every day, twice a week may be satisfactory. And if the woman would prefer to have sex once a week, twice a week may be doable. In this case, both partners in a relationship may be satisfied with their sexual frequency. The problem comes when there is no middle ground, compromise, or communication.

THE BENEFITS OF TOUCH

The largest organ in your body is your skin. Physical contact and touch is very important to your physical and emotional well-being. Many studies have shown the importance of touch. Premature infants who were touched more gained more weight, were more alert and active, and left the hospital earlier than those premature infants who were given standard care.[3] Even adults need to be touched. Massage, which is basically a form of touch, has been shown to reduce pain, diminish depression, facilitate growth, and enhance the immune function.[4]

Of course, what is sex but an intense and intimate form of touch? When else do you get this amount of skin-to-skin contact? Think of all the ways touch makes you feel better: a hug, holding hands, massage, cuddling, kissing, and sex. Notice how those who are relatively isolated feel a need to be touched. Touch is a basic human need. Think how close you feel to someone when you have that much of your body touching another while being sexually intimate. That's one of the main reasons sex is so pleasurable.

VIAGRA IN WOMEN

Some of you may say, "I know all of this but the problem is I just can't seem to get in the mood. Is there something I can take to help?" There is an increased interest in the use of testosterone and sildenafil (Viagra) in women to help with low libido. Viagra use in women has shown mixed results.

Viagra works by increasing blood flow to the genital area. In men, the improved blood flow into the penis causes an erection, which is why it's so successful in helping men. In women, increased blood flow to the genital area does . . . what? The data on the use of Viagra in women are limited and it is unclear whether it helps with sexual desire. This is not surprising because increasing blood flow to the genitals does not change the way your brain works.

Viagra can have side effects including headache, flushing, upset stomach, bluish or blurred vision, and rarely heart attack or stroke. Anyone taking medications containing nitrates such as nitroglycerin should not take Viagra under any circumstances.

The bottom line? There is no easy answer to decreased sex drive. This issue is affected by a complex interplay of psychological, emotional, and hormonal factors. The best any of us can hope to do is to work toward a loving relationship and find a balance of all these elements.

HORMONES AND SEX

Hormonal changes may also contribute to a drop in your sex drive. A woman's fertility decreases significantly in her midthirties. At the cellular level, the ovary begins to undergo changes with a progressive deterioration in the production of the eggs and hormones. This decline in ovarian function may be subtle in its manifestation, but may be what contributes to the decrease in libido and the increase in premenstrual symptoms during perimenopause.

Mood Swings

These hormonal changes can increase irritability, which may also contribute to tension in your relationship with your significant other. Fatigue and stress compound this problem. The people closest to you may feel the brunt of this. You may look at your significant other and actually wonder why he has changed. "When did my husband become so irritating?" What you used to think of as cute or quirky may now seem irritating and bothersome.

Maybe your significant other did change. And perhaps so did you. And as you both evolved, so did your relationship. You can't remain in that initial love-at-first-sight stage forever. But unless you keep the lines of communication open and spend quality time together, you may end up growing apart and not realize this until it's too late.

Estrogen's Role in Sex

As we have already noted, hormones may play a role in this. Estrogen may have a more direct effect on sexual functioning. Declining estrogen levels cause a decrease in the amount of vaginal lubrication during arousal, thinning of the vaginal lining, and less blood flow to the genital area, which may affect sensation in the genital area. The vagina becomes less elastic and less accommodating during intercourse, which along with less lubrication, can lead to painful intercourse. Pain with intercourse will definitely affect your sex drive.

Nonetheless, estrogen seems to play a minimal direct role in sexual desire.[5] The effects of estrogen on desire mostly seem to be through indirect mechanisms as described above.

PMS

PMS also seems to worsen during perimenopause. (This is described in more detail in chapter 4.) The increasing moodiness and irritability in the week or two before your period can definitely have a negative influence on your sex drive. You may actually notice an improvement in your libido the week after your period until midcycle when you ovulate, then a decrease the weeks before your next period. How much of this is directly related to hormones is unclear. But there is some sort of hormonal connection that does influence your sex drive in relation to your menstrual cycle.

Testosterone in Women

Women's bodies make testosterone, the male hormone that plays a role in your sex drive, building up your bones and muscles, and feelings of general well-being. A large portion of the testosterone in a woman is produced by the ovaries. As you grow older, your testosterone levels gradually decrease. Testosterone levels in women at forty are about half those of women in their early twenties.[6]

Some people feel that a low level of testosterone contributes to a low sex drive. This is most clearly seen in younger women who have had both their ovaries removed. These women have about a 50 percent drop in male hormone levels and a significant drop in their libido.[7] Giving them testosterone has been shown to improve their libido, which supports the notion that testosterone plays an important role in sexual desire.[8]

However, in healthy premenopausal women who still have their ovaries, the relation between testosterone and sexual desire is less clear. Studies have shown inconsistent results between testosterone levels and sexual desire. Women with and without a diagnosis of hypoactive sexual desire (a very low sex drive) had no significant difference in testosterone levels.[9] So while testosterone may influence sexual desire, testosterone alone is not enough for women to experience sexual desire.

One major problem with studying male hormones such as testosterone in women is that the accuracy of testosterone tests has been found to be lacking and that "normal" testosterone levels in women of different ages are unknown.[10] Another source of confusion is a significant placebo response in treating these problems.

Testosterone: The Magic Pill?

As noted, testosterone has improved sexual functioning and psychological well-being in women who have had their ovaries removed. Similarly, testosterone may be beneficial for women whose ovaries have been rendered nonfunctional by radiation (usually in women treated for cancer).

The results of testosterone use in other women is not so clear. Some women are diagnosed with a testosterone deficiency, which is measured by checking a free testosterone level. A free testosterone level shows the amount of testosterone that is not bound to a protein in blood. This free testosterone is the form that is biologically active. These women with low free testosterone levels who are having problems with loss of libido may benefit from testosterone therapy though the evidence for its effectiveness is currently very weak.[11]

Side Effects of Testosterone

However, testosterone has side effects including increased hair growth on the face and chest, hair loss from the head, acne, oily skin, deepening of the voice, bloating, fluid retention, and liver problems. Testosterone may also have a negative effect on cholesterol levels and the heart.[12] All of these side effects are generally reversible once the testosterone is discontinued except for the deepening of the voice. So if you are a singer, realize that there can be a permanent deepening of your voice if you use testosterone.

Testosterone can be given as a pill, a patch, a cream, an injection, or as an implant. To date, neither the optimal route by which to give testosterone nor the dose has been determined. If you, under a physician's guidance, choose to use testosterone, by whatever means the testosterone is given, testosterone levels should be checked to make sure that you are not getting too high a dose, as higher doses tend to lead to more side effects.

PERCEIVED LOSS OF ATTRACTIVENESS

Physical changes can lead to a perceived loss of attractiveness and may bring about a decrease in sexual desire. During perimenopause and menopause, many women experience physical alterations: graying hair, wrinkles, increasing weight, and loss of skin tone. These physical changes mark another time of transition. During puberty, those physical changes such as breast development, hair growth, and menstrual cycles signaled your passage from a child to an adult. Now, these physical changes are sometimes associated with leaving a younger stage of adulthood and entering a more mature phase of life. For some women, this transition is difficult because of our culture's worship of thin, youthful beauty.

The Media's Effect

In the American culture of the new millennium, we have been trained to view thin, young women as the ideal, as the definition of attractiveness and beauty. Look at Marilyn Monroe. She was the symbol of beauty of her time and she had a much fuller figure than most movie stars today. Perhaps if she were an actress today, her producer might be asking her to lose some weight to better fit in with the modern definition of beauty. Much of how we determine what is beautiful is driven by the media.

Consider this. Women in Fiji are plump. They have been that way for generations and the men and women liked it that way. Eating disorders were rare. But after 1995, increasing numbers of young women started dieting, trying to stay thinner.[13] And eating disorders became more prevalent, especially among teenagers. What changed? Through the wonders of modern technology and satellite communication, *Melrose Place*, *Beverly Hills 90210*, and other Western shows and movies were beamed to Fiji starting in 1995. Thus, a change in their perception of beauty occurred.

So the media has a powerful influence on our perception of beauty and attractiveness. It is uncommon to see a woman in her forties and fifties portrayed as a beautiful, sexy character. Sexuality and youth are so often intertwined that a common misperception is that older people aren't interested in sex, or don't have sex. Women then look at their changing bodies and may feel unattractive. This may even be an unconscious feeling that can have a negative impact on their sex drive.

Women who are self-confident and who are comfortable with who they are can enjoy their sexuality. They know that sexual desire in a man is not

Figure 6.3

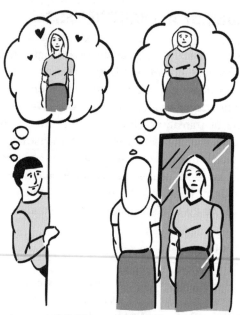

always dependant on youthful beauty. Feeling sensuous and confident add to a woman's allure. And don't forget that men age in appearance, too. Few men can retain the looks of Sean Connery through their lifetimes. Moreover, as a relationship matures, sex becomes a form of communication, a way to share love and intimacy that transcends the media model of sexuality.

HEALTH PROBLEMS

For those of you who enjoy relatively good health, you simply need to make more time for your partner. For others, as they get older, they find that health problems become more common. Exercise can improve your health and self-image, which may have a positive impact on your sex drive.

Unfortunately, you may develop health problems despite your best efforts and that may interfere with your sex drive. Leaking urine (urinary incontinence) becomes more common as you get older. Some women may leak urine during sex or with orgasm. Because of the embarrassment, many women with this problem avoid intercourse. (See chapter 2 for more information about urinary incontinence.) In addition, yeast infections may cause irritation and pain with intercourse. Other medical problems may cause fatigue and loss of energy, which may also affect your libido. By treating the health problems, you may also improve your libido.

Medications

Certain medications can cause a decrease in your sex drive. Birth control pills and other hormonal forms of contraception can actually decrease sexual desire in some women. The class of antidepressants know as selective serotonin reuptake inhibitor (SSRIs) such as fluoxetine (Prozac), paroxetine (Paxil), sertraline (Zoloft), venlafaxine (Effexor) and others are all known to potentially decrease sex drive and may also affect your ability to have orgasm. Other antidepressants and antipsychotic medications can also decrease sexual desire, lubrication, and orgasm.

Hormones, including birth control pills, estrogen therapy for menopausal symptoms, and tamoxifen, can affect sexual desire in some women. Antihistamines can decrease vaginal lubrication.[14]

If possible, you may want to change your medications, or go to a lower dose to see if your sex drive returns. Some women notice fewer problems when they switch between different antidepressants, especially if they go to a different class of antidepressants. Changing hormones and adding testosterone may help some women with their libido. Do not discontinue or change the dosage of your medications without advice from your physician.

Decreased Lubrication

> *At forty-two years old, I am not sure if I am premenopausal. Should I feel something different at this age? One thing does come to mind, for the first time in my life, I am aware of my vagina. The awareness is a feeling of dryness. Maybe, the KY jelly my sister gave me for my fortieth birthday should not have been tossed out.*
>
> *—Pam Cray*

Decreasing estrogen levels lead to a decrease in the amount of lubrication you make when you become aroused. It may take longer to become lubricated and the quality of your lubrication may change as you go through menopause. The vaginal dryness that results can cause discomfort or pain with intercourse, especially when your partner first enters you.

Not all women will have problems related to these vaginal changes. Using a lubricant during intercourse for some women is all that is needed to help with the dryness and discomfort. Vaginal lubricants can be purchased without a prescription. Water-based lubricants such as Astroglide and KY Jelly are the best. They can be liberally reapplied as needed.

Astroglide and KY Jelly are glycerine-based lubricants that do not dry out quickly and can be rewetted with water or saliva. Oil-based lubricants, and those containing coloring or perfumes, should be avoided because they can irritate the vaginal walls or weaken latex condoms.[15]

If Lubricants Don't Help

However, even with the use of lubricants, some women still experience discomfort with intercourse. Part of the reason may be the changes that occur in the vagina as estrogen levels drop. The vagina becomes narrower, shorter, and less elastic. This makes it less accommodating to your partner and more uncomfortable for you.

Sex may also be more uncomfortable because the vaginal walls are thinner and more likely to be irritated through the friction of intercourse. This, along with the decreased elasticity of the vaginal walls, may cause the vaginal walls to tear with intercourse, leading to pain and bleeding.

As you become aroused, changes occur in your vagina: there is an increase in blood flow to your genitals and the vagina opens, elongates, and becomes lubricated in anticipation of intercourse. However, with the lower levels of estrogen seen after menopause, the vaginal response during arousal is reduced, potentially leading to discomfort.

If lubricants don't help, the main option is estrogen. Estrogen helps with lubrication, thickens the vaginal walls and makes them more elastic, and improves blood flow to the genital area. Estrogen can be given either locally as a cream, ring, or tablet in the vagina, or systemically as a pill, patch, injection, or pellet. However, estrogen can be absorbed through the vaginal walls, sometimes to a significant degree and can go to the rest of the body. (For the other benefits and risks of estrogen, please refer to chapter 9.)

Decreased Genital Sensation

Some women notice a decrease in sensation in the genital area as they get older. Part of this change, as noted, may be due to the loss of estrogen. As estrogen levels drop, there is less blood flow to the genital area and changes occur in the vaginal walls that may alter sensation in that area.

Part of the loss in sensation may also have resulted from injury to nerves in the vaginal area due to childbirth. As your baby came through the birth canal, nerves to the pelvis were stretched and possibly injured, and this may still be affecting you. Not only can this affect your sex life, it can also make it more likely for you to have problems such as urinary incontinence. Estrogen may help somewhat, but if the diminished sensations are due to nerve injury, not much can be done at this time.

Medical problems such as multiple sclerosis and surgical procedures can also cause nerve damage and may impact sensation and orgasm.

PAINFUL INTERCOURSE

Pain with intercourse can be caused by a number of reasons. Pain can occur near the opening of the vagina when your partner first enters you. Or the pain can be deep inside where you feel like your partner is hitting something inside of you. Or you may have no pain during intercourse, but hurt afterward.

A lack of lubrication and vaginal changes described above can cause pain. A number of conditions, such as lichen sclerosis, a skin condition, become more common after menopause, and can cause irritation and pain around the vaginal opening. The key to helping with this problem is getting a proper diagnosis, which may require a biopsy where a piece of tissue is pinched off and sent to the lab for evaluation.

Vaginismus

Sometimes you can have a condition called vaginismus where the muscles around the opening to the vagina become so tight that intercourse becomes painful. If you have intercourse and it's painful, no matter what the reason (lack of lubrication, vaginal infections, large penis size, rough sex, or any other reason), you may be more hesitant about sex the next time. Your body doesn't like pain and tries to protect itself against anything that might hurt. If intercourse hurts, then your body tries to keep things out of the vagina by tightening the muscles around the opening. But if you still have intercourse, it hurts when your partner pushes through those tightened muscles. This then leads to a vicious cycle: when you have intercourse, it hurts, so your body tightens up more, and when you have intercourse again, it hurts more.

Vaginal Dilators

Treatment options for vaginismus include the use of vaginal dilators. The concept behind their use is to get your vagina used to the idea that something can enter it without causing pain. You can use medically approved vaginal dilators or you can use tapered candles in graded sizes from the smallest (about the size of your index finger) to the largest (the size of your partner's penis), with two or three sizes in between. Pick a time when you won't be disturbed. Cover the smallest candle with a condom, lubricate it with a water based lubricant such as Astroglide, and then slowly insert it into your vagina. Once the dilator is inside the vagina, tighten the pelvic floor muscles (by doing Kegel's exercises described in chapter 2) around the dilator and then relax. Continue to tighten and relax the pelvic floor muscles around the dilator for several minutes, then remove the dilator.

Do this daily until you feel no discomfort when inserting the smallest dilator for a week. Then move to the next largest dilator and repeat the previous steps. Keep working your way up until you are using the largest dilator without any discomfort. During this time, do not attempt to have any vaginal intercourse with your partner. If you do before you have made it to the largest dilator, it may cause pain and rekindle the vaginismus. By tightening your pelvic muscles, you also learn to relax them so that they won't be so tense when you finally have vaginal intercourse.

Once you are using the largest dilator without problem, you may then try vaginal intercourse with your partner. A glass of wine (if it doesn't interfere with your medications) may help you relax. Use a position where you can control the speed and depth of penetration. You will also want to make sure you are well lubricated, either with your own fluids or with a lubricant. If you feel some discomfort, stop, then tighten and relax the pelvic floor, which may allow you to let your partner deeper inside. Keep doing this until your partner is completely inside. At that point, tighten and relax again as you get used to this. If you are doing well at this point, you can slowly start to move and reexplore that ageless intimate dance of love.

Deep Pain with Intercourse

Sometimes, the pain with sex may feel deeper, as if your partner is hitting something deep inside of you. This could be caused by the size of your partner's penis, how your uterus is positioned in the pelvis, or it could be a sign of other problems such as endometriosis, adenomyosis, or fibroids.

Endometriosis

Endometriosis is a condition in which the endometrium, or the lining of the uterus, grows outside of the uterus—where it's not supposed to be. Endometriosis causes inflammation and pain. The most common areas for endometriosis to grow are behind the uterus and around the ovaries. Endometriosis usually causes the most pain right before and during your period. Endometriosis can also cause pain with intercourse. Think about it—if your pelvis is inflamed and irritated and your partner starts poking and prodding with his penis in that sensitive area, it's going to hurt.

Diagnosis of Endometriosis

Unfortunately, the only way to tell if you have endometriosis is through surgery. Blood tests, ultrasound, CT scans, and other imaging studies cannot detect endometriosis. The endometriosis has to be seen to be diagnosed and the main way to see the endometriosis is to look inside your body with a laparoscope.

Laparoscopy is an outpatient surgical procedure where a laparoscope, a telescope-like instrument, is placed into your belly so that the inside of your abdomen and pelvis can be seen. If endometriosis is seen, it can be vaporized with a laser, burned with electrical cautery, or cut out and removed. However, most of the time, the endometriosis eventually comes back.

Treatment of Endometriosis

You don't necessarily have to have surgery to treat the pain, however. Usually, laparoscopy is done after other therapies have failed. Other forms of treatment include the use of anti-inflammatory medications such as ibuprofen or naproxen as well as hormonal options. Birth control pills and progestins (synthetic compounds that act like progesterone) can suppress endometriosis and can be used long term.

GnRH agonists such as Depo-Lupron shut down the ovaries, leading to a temporary menopausal state. Estrogen stimulates endometriosis to grow. By shutting down the ovaries, estrogen levels drop, and the endometriosis becomes inactive. However, GnRH agonists are used for only six to twelve months because they do cause some bone loss. (See chapter 3 for more information about GnRH agonists.)

Hysterectomy is sometimes used to treat endometriosis. However, if the ovaries are left behind, the endometriosis may continue to grow and cause pain. Removing the ovaries at the time of the hysterectomy is very effective at treating endometriosis, but also puts you through menopause and has other potential downsides (see chapter 3).

Once you have gone through menopause and estrogen levels have dropped, endometriosis usually resolves and is no longer a problem—another benefit of menopause.

> ***The "hot sweats" during the night times are minor compared to the years of painful menstrual cramps.***
> ***—Linda O'Connell***

Estrogen therapy after your ovaries are removed or after natural menopause can sometimes cause the endometriosis to recur. Remember, estrogen stimulates the endometriosis to grow. Usually, the low doses of estrogen used after menopause will not stimulate the endometriosis, however, and if you are having severe menopausal symptoms, estrogen is a reasonable option.

Adenomyosis

Adenomyosis is a condition in which the endometrium grows deep inside the wall of the uterus. Adenomyosis can lead to several problems including worsening cramping, heavier periods, and pain deep in the pelvis with intercourse. Adenomyosis is treated similarly to endometriosis with anti-inflammatory medications used first, then hormonal remedies, and finally surgery. (See chapter 3 for more information about adenomyosis.)

Fibroids

Fibroids are a common finding in women and usually don't cause any problems. If they get very large, fibroids can cause bleeding, pelvic pressure, and pain. Treatment options include myomectomy (removing the fibroids), uterine artery embolization, and hysterectomy. (See chapter 3 for more information on fibroids and their treatment.)

DIFFICULTY ACHIEVING ORGASM

Orgasm is characterized by a peak in sexual pleasure that is accompanied by rhythmic contractions of the genital and reproductive organs, cardiovascular and respiratory changes, and a release of sexual tension.[16] Difficulties with orgasm are not uncommon. About 10 percent of women have never had an orgasm and at least 50 percent of women report situational or intermittent orgasmic problems.[17] Many women do not have orgasm as a result of only vaginal intercourse. They need more stimulation, either manual, oral, or mechanical, to help them achieve orgasm.

Lack of knowledge and sexual inexperience can lead to the problem of difficulty achieving orgasm. Sexual inhibitions related to feelings of guilt, anxiety, or past history of sexual abuse or trauma can also affect a woman's ability to have orgasm. Some women have "performance anxiety" where they feel pressured to have an orgasm by their partner. Relationship problems with the partner can also cause difficulty with orgasm. Negative feelings can suppress a woman's ability to have orgasm even when there is sufficient stimulation. Medications such as antidepressants may also affect the ability to achieve orgasm.

Lest we seem to put too much emphasis on this, orgasm is but one aspect of intercourse that determines a woman's satisfaction with sex. Sex can be pleasurable and satisfying for women even without orgasm. The same is not true for men. Orgasm is their goal and without orgasm, men feel sexually unfulfilled. This may explain why a woman's lack of orgasm can be distressing to her partner. Some men want the woman to be fully satisfied with the sexual experience and in the man's eyes, that means orgasm. Other men feel that they are inadequately meeting the sexual needs of their partner if she does not have an orgasm.

But whether you have an orgasm or not, it is most important that you feel content with your situation. You are not doing this for your partner. If you wish to pursue this further, treatment options depend on the cause of the problem. If it is a matter of inadequate knowledge and/or stimulation, books are available to help you learn about your body and techniques to improve stimulation so that you are able to achieve orgasm. If the problem is related to sexual inhibitions, especially those caused by history of abuse or relationship problems, therapy can be helpful. Therapy and/or books can also be helpful at reducing guilt or anxiety and accepting your normal sexual feelings.

It's ironic that in this culture of overt sexuality, a double standard still to some degree exists while sexual images bombard us from all sides. Getting beyond this double message can take many years for some women, leaving some never comfortable with their sexuality. This not only affects orgasm, but sexual desire and arousal as well.

THE BOTTOM LINE

Sex is an important and natural part of a relationship. Menopause does not mean the end of sex or sexual desire. The most important factor determining sexual functioning after menopause is your level of sexual functioning before menopause. For most couples, menopause itself does not significantly affect their sexual relationship. True, perimenopause and menopause can lead to changes that impact sexual functioning, but most women continue to have a healthy sex life as they age.

Unfortunately, there is no magic pill you can take to increase your libido. No easy answer is available to address this problem. Open communication, time, and effort are needed to improve this part of your relationship. For so long, your sex life and sexual drive was taken for granted. Only when there is a change do you take notice. Like anything else worth doing, your sex life also needs to be worked on to make it a vibrant part of your life. When there is communication and understanding, you and your partner adapt to each other's changes, maintaining and even strengthening your bond.

CHAPTER 7

I CAN'T BE PREGNANT...

*I*f you're now in your late thirties or forties, you may not be planning to have children or any more children. Yet, for some of you, the use of birth control has become intermittent or nonexistent. You rationalize that your fertility is minimal, you and/or your partner don't like condoms, and the pill makes you bloated, so you figure you'll just take your chances. Just like a teenager.

That is, until one night, lying in bed, you realize your period is late. And then you panic while trying to find a twenty-four-hour pharmacy to buy a pregnancy test. You rationalize that it's just an irregularity in your cycle. You've heard this happens as you get closer to menopause. But until you've gotten the results from a pregnancy test, you've already gone through a million scenarios of what a baby in your life at this time would mean.

There is a significant decline in fertility after age thirty-five and even more so after forty. Some women feel that they don't have to worry as much about contraception because of this, so they prematurely discontinue its use. Moreover, they may not find any of the birth control choices particularly attractive, for various reasons, such as past difficulties (the shot made me gain so much weight), personal dislikes (I just don't like the feel of condoms), and/or concerns about possible risks and side effects (I heard the pill can cause cancer). Does this type of thinking sound familiar? If you've been around teenagers, you'll hear similar sentiments: "It can't happen to me." "Condoms are icky." "The pill made Allison blow up like a whale."

UNINTENDED PREGNANCIES

By the time most women have reached their forties, they no longer plan to have any more children. However, the highest rates of unintended pregnancies occurs in the teens *and in the forties*. Data from the National Survey of Family Growth reveals that 51 percent of pregnancies in women over the age of forty were unintended. Of these unintended pregnancies, 65 percent ended in abortion.[1] This highlights the inadequacy of contraceptive use in women in general of this age group.

The most common form of birth control in women over thirty is female sterilization. In a 1995 survey, 36 percent of women between forty and forty-four had undergone sterilization.[2] Fifteen percent of their partners had a vasectomy and 9 percent used condoms. Only 4 percent used birth control pills; other methods were used to an even lesser degree.

Here is a list of birth control options and their ideal effectiveness versus real-world effectiveness in order of effectiveness with typical use:[3]

Birth control method	Lowest expected rate of pregnancy if used perfectly over one year (%)	Rate of pregnancy with typical use over one year (%)
No method	85	85
Sponge: Never had a baby	6.0	18.0
Sponge: Had a baby	9.0	28.0
Spermicides	3.0	21.0
Diaphragm and spermicide	6.0	18.0
Cervical cap	6.0	18.0
Rhythm Method	1 to 9	20
Withdrawal	4.0	18.0
Condom	2.0	12.0
Progestin-only pill (Minipill)	0.5	3.0
Combination pill	0.1	3.0
Depo-Provera	0.3	0.3
Norplant	0.2	0.2
IUD (Copper T 380A)	0.8	<1.0
Tubal ligation	0.2	0.4
Vasectomy	0.1	0.15

Here is a list of birth control options available to you and your partner:

- Condom
- Diaphragm
- Cervical cap
- Female condom
- Contraceptive jelly, sponge
- Periodic abstinence (rhythm method, natural family planning)
- Withdrawal (coitus interruptus)
- Oral contraceptive (birth control pills)
- Contraceptive ring
- Contraceptive patch
- Morning-after pill (emergency contraception)
- Lunelle (the one-month shot)
- Depo-provera (the three-month shot)
- Norplant (which is currently not on the market but may be re-released in the future)
- Intrauterine devices
- Tubal ligation
- Vasectomy
- Abstinence

So many choices. Let us review the different methods and their advantages and disadvantages to help you come to your decision.

CONDOMS

Tried and true, condoms have been around for centuries. Since the 1930s latex condoms have been available, but their use declined in the 1960s and 1970s when other effective forms of birth control became available. The fear of HIV and other sexually transmitted diseases renewed interest in condoms in the 1980s. For perimenopausal women, condoms provide relatively effective contraception.

Condoms often get a bum rap because they are associated more with younger people and are seen as a less sophisticated form of birth control. Many men and women don't like the way condoms feel. I sometimes hear: "My husband/boyfriend won't wear one." Remember, you could always offer abstinence as an alternative.

Condoms are an effective form of birth control with many benefits and a few minor side effects.

The advantages of condoms:

- Prevent the spread of several sexually transmitted diseases (but not all)
- Easy to use
- Used only when needed
- Few risks or side effects
- Can be bought without a prescription
- Relatively inexpensive
- Readily available

There are some downsides to condoms:

- Latex can be irritating
- Some people are allergic to latex
- Not as effective in preventing pregnancy as some other forms of birth control
- Decreases sensitivity in men (which may or may not be a downside)
- Some men and women dislike the way it feels
- May be more difficult to maintain adequate lubrication

Condoms: "Safer Sex"

Condoms are associated with "safe sex," which gives some people a false sense of security. They feel that the use of condoms provides them with a bulletproof shield against sexually transmitted diseases. Though condoms are good at protecting women against some diseases like gonorrhea, chlamydia, trichomonas, and HIV, they unfortunately offer less protection against herpes, human papillomavirus (the virus that causes genital warts and abnormal pap smears), molluscum contagiosum (a viral infection that causes smooth growths up to several millimeters across in the genital area), the Hepatitis B virus, syphilis, and pubic lice.

Though condoms do not protect you against several sexually transmitted infections, they provide more protection than any other form of birth control and protection similar to that of the female condom. Your only true protection against all sexually transmitted infections is to avoid genital-to-

Figure 7.1

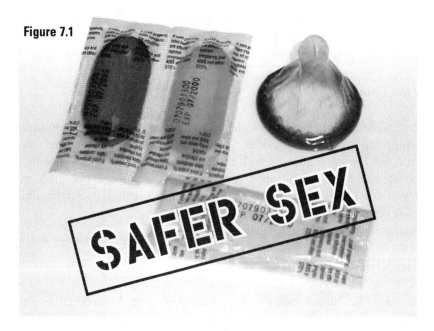

genital or oral-to-genital contact. Even if there is no penetration, some of these infections can still be transmitted.

Types of Condoms

There are three types of condoms: latex, polyurethane, and natural. Latex condoms are made from latex, a compound extracted from *Hevea brasiliensis* or rubber trees. Polyurethane is a plastic compound used to make some condoms. Natural condoms are made from animal sources. Polyurethane and natural condoms can be used if one of the partners is allergic to latex. *However, natural condoms do not necessarily prevent the transmission of HIV.* Natural condoms have tiny holes, too small for sperm to pass through, but large enough for the tiny HIV virus to pass.

Lubricants and Condoms

If you use a condom and lubricant when having intercourse, use only water-based lubricants such as Astroglide or KY Jelly. Oil-based lubricants such as Vaseline, baby oil, massage oils, cooking oils, mineral oils, body lotions, suntan oils and lotions, butter, margarine, shortening, and even whipped cream can damage the latex. This increases the chance that the condom will break.

Condoms need to be worn before there is any contact of the penis with the vagina. Even before ejaculation some semen containing thousands of sperm leaks out of the urethra. Only one is needed to fertilize the egg.

If the Condom Breaks

If a condom breaks before ejaculation and during intercourse, stop immediately and replace the condom. If it breaks after your partner has ejaculated, wash away the semen with soap and water, though it may already be too late because within seconds, sperm have already made it into the uterus. If you don't already have the morning-after pill, contact your physician about obtaining it.

DIAPHRAGM

Another oldie, but not such a goodie, is the diaphragm. A diaphragm is not as effective as other forms of contraception. Because of the decreasing fertility during perimenopause, however, a diaphragm is not unreasonable to use and has no hormonal side effects. A diaphragm is made of latex and looks like a tennis ball cut in half. A metal ring on the edge of the diaphragm holds it open and in place in the vagina. The diaphragm works by blocking the sperm from reaching the cervix. However, the diaphragm cannot completely seal the vagina, so sperm can slip past its edge. Spermicide helps improve the effectiveness of the diaphragm, but even then it is less effective than condoms.

The advantages of the diaphragm:

- Used only when needed
- Few risks or side effects
- Offers some protection against pelvic infections
- Relatively inexpensive
- Under a woman's control

Disadvantages of diaphragm:

- Latex can be irritating
- Some people are allergic to latex
- May increase bladder infections

- Available only with a prescription
- Not as effective in preventing pregnancy as some other forms of birth control
- More difficult to use than other forms of birth control
- Some women are uncomfortable with inserting the diaphragm
- Some feel it decreases the spontaneity of sex
- Some feel it decreases sensitivity

A diaphragm is more difficult to use than most other forms of birth control. It requires some manual dexterity to place in the proper location and to remove. The diaphragm should be left in place for six hours after intercourse, but no more than twenty-four hours. If you have intercourse again within that twenty-four-hour period, you should use additional spermicide in the vagina each time you have intercourse.

CERVICAL CAP

The cervical cap is a barrier form of birth control, which works similarly to the diaphragm and has similar advantages. The cervical cap is fitted over the cervix to block the sperm from getting to the cervix. It is about as effective as the diaphragm. It can be used with or without spermicide, but spermicide increases its effectiveness.

The advantages of the cervical cap are basically the same as the diaphragm. However, it can be left in place for up to forty-eight hours (as opposed to the twenty-four hours for the diaphragm).

Disadvantages of the cervical cap:

- Latex can be irritating
- Some people are allergic to latex
- Available only with a prescription
- Not as effective in preventing pregnancy as other forms of birth control
- More difficult to use than other forms of birth control
- May cause a bad-smelling discharge, especially if left in for over twenty-four hours
- Some women are uncomfortable with inserting the cervical cap
- Some feel it decreases the spontaneity of sex
- May be dislodged from the cervix during intercourse

The cervical cap is more difficult to use than most other forms of birth control. It requires some manual dexterity to place the cap in the proper location, and also to remove it. You have to be able to identify the cervix and place the cap correctly over it. Each time after intercourse, the cap needs to be checked to see if the cervix is still covered. The cap should be left in place for eight hours after intercourse, and can be left in place up to forty-eight hours. If you have intercourse again within that forty-eight-hour period, you should use additional spermicide in the vagina each time you have intercourse.

FEMALE CONDOM

The female condom is a barrier form of birth control that uses a polyurethane pouch to line the vagina. The pouch has a ring at the bottom which is placed over the cervix. A ring at the opening of the pouch stays outside of the vagina. The pouch is lubricated with silicone and catches the sperm.

The advantages of the female condom:

- Used only when needed
- Few risks or side effects
- Helps protect against sexually transmitted diseases
- Under a woman's control
- Does not require a prescription

Disadvantages of the female condom:

- Cumbersome to use
- Relatively expensive
- Not as effective in preventing pregnancy as some other forms of birth control
- Some women are uncomfortable with inserting the female condom
- Some feel it decreases the spontaneity of sex

CONTRACEPTIVE SPONGE

The contraceptive sponge is made up of a sponge containing spermicide. The sponge is placed in the vagina prior to any penetration and is effective for twenty-four hours. It is more effective than foam, jelly, and tablet spermicides but not as effective as the diaphragm or condom. It works by killing the sperm, but it also blocks the cervix somewhat and absorbs the semen.

The advantages of the contraceptive sponge:

- Used only when needed
- Few risks or side effects
- Relatively inexpensive
- Under a woman's control
- Can be left in place for up to twenty-four hours
- Does not require a prescription
- Less messy than other spermicides

The disadvantages of the sponge:

- Can be irritating
- Can cause allergic reaction
- Can cause vaginal dryness and irritation
- Not as effective in preventing pregnancy as some other forms of birth control
- Some women are uncomfortable with inserting the sponge
- Some feel it decreases the spontaneity of sex
- Difficult to obtain in the United States

SPERMICIDES

Spermicides are chemicals used in the vagina to kill sperm. Spermicides can come in jellies, foams, suppositories, or creams. The spermicide should be placed *before* any penetration and reapplied each time you have intercourse. If you have intercourse several times in one night, you should reapply the spermicide each time. Applying the spermicide or douching after intercourse is too late and will not work. Within seconds, sperm have already passed through the cervical canal into the uterus.

The advantages of spermicides:

- Used only when needed
- Few risks or side effects

- Relatively inexpensive
- Under a woman's control
- Simple to use
- Does not require a prescription

The disadvantages of spermicides:

- Can be irritating
- Can cause allergic reaction
- Not as effective in preventing pregnancy as some other forms of birth control
- Some feel it decreases the spontaneity of sex
- Can be messy
- Skin irritation can lead to breaks in the skin that can *increase* the risk of acquiring HIV

NATURAL FAMILY PLANNING (RHYTHM METHOD)

Natural family planning or the rhythm method is a method of birth control that relies on avoiding intercourse when pregnancy may occur. The sperm may live for up to seven days after intercourse in your body. After ovulation when the egg is released from the ovary, it has a one- to two-day window when it can be fertilized. So the time to avoid intercourse is roughly seven days before ovulation to two days after.

The main question is, When does ovulation occur? Typically, you ovulate about fourteen days before your next cycle. Of course, if you have to wait until your next cycle to figure this out, it's already too late. If your cycles are very regular, you can subtract fourteen days from your cycle to estimate when you would ovulate.

For example, if your cycles are thirty days apart, you subtract fourteen from thirty to get sixteen. You would then know that you ovulate around day sixteen of your cycle, counting the first day that you bleed as day one of your cycle. However, this gives you only an estimate of when you ovulate and works only if your cycles are very regular.

Length of cycle in days	26	27	28	29	30	31	32
Estimated time of ovulation	Day 12	13	14	15	16	17	18

For the calendar method, you follow six cycles and record the length of each cycle. Subtract eighteen days from the length of the shortest cycle to calculate the beginning of your fertile period. Subtract eleven from the length of the longest cycle to determine the end of your fertile period. For example, if your cycles run from twenty-eight to thirty days apart, your fertile time would start on day ten of your cycle and go to day nineteen of your cycle, ten days a month when you would have to abstain or use another form of birth control.[4]

Carefully observing the cervical mucus also gives an indication of the fertile time period. When the cervical mucus turns sticky, slippery, and wet, this is a sign that ovulation is going to occur soon. Avoiding intercourse during this time until the fourth day after the mucus returns to normal is another way to attempt to time intercourse.[5]

Many times, women use a combination of these and other methods to determine their fertile period. However, this works only if the menstrual cycles are regular. Not every woman's body works according to clockwork. Moreover, the problem with a woman going through perimenopause is that cycles often become irregular. Irregular cycles will make it impossible to determine when ovulation will occur, thus increasing the likelihood of failure and possible pregnancy.

WITHDRAWAL (COITUS INTERRUPTUS)

Withdrawal, pulling out before ejaculation, is another less effective form of birth control. The theory is that if the male pulls out before ejaculation, no sperm is deposited in the vagina. The main problem is that before ejaculation, a small amount of semen leaks out, containing thousands of sperm—and that's enough to fertilize the egg and cause pregnancy. That's the reason for the old joke, "What do you call a woman who's using withdrawal for birth control? Pregnant." The other problem is having your partner withdraw before he starts ejaculating. Although it has its faults and does not provide protection against sexually transmitted infections, withdrawal appears to be almost as effective as the diaphragm and cervical cap. This is because some sperm can slip past diaphragms and cervical caps, perhaps similar to the amount of sperm that leaks out before ejaculation.

ORAL CONTRACEPTIVES (BIRTH CONTROL PILLS)

Birth control pills (also known as "The Pill") are the most common form of contraception, used by over 80 percent of women in the United States at some point in their lives.[6] Many women are under the impression that the pill is unsafe after the age of thirty-five. Birth control pills not only offer reliable contraception, but also offer other noncontraceptive benefits in perimenopausal women, such as cycle control.

However, there is a dramatic decrease in oral contraceptive use with age. Though most women have used birth control pills, myths and/or misunderstandings about the risks of the pill persist. "It will make you fat." "The Pill causes cancer." "It can cause heart attacks or strokes if you're over thirty-five." Let's explore further and separate fact from fiction.

How Does the Birth Control Pill Work?

Most birth control pills contain the female hormones estrogen and progestins (synthetic forms of the female hormone progesterone). These pills are also referred to as "combination birth control pills" or "combination oral contraceptives," referring to the combination of estrogen and progestins in one pill. Progestin-only pills are generally referred to as "minipills."

When a woman takes birth control pills, the pituitary gland senses plenty of estrogen and progesterone, so it does not stimulate the ovary. The ovary therefore does not produce an egg. The progestins also thicken the cervical mucus, making it harder for the sperm to pass through this area, and change the lining of the uterus, which hinders implantation.

Why Is There a Concern in Using Birth Controll Pills in Women over Thirty-Five?

In the past and even now, physicians have been reluctant to prescribe birth control pills for women over the age of thirty-five. Concerns over increased risks of heart attacks and strokes in these women prompted this attitude. When birth control pills first came out in the 1960s, studies showed that women over the age of thirty-five who used these pills had a significantly higher risk of dying from a heart attack or having a stroke.[7]

However, after reanalyzing the studies, these risks were seen only in women over the age of thirty-five who smoked or had other risk factors for cardiovascular disease such as diabetes or high blood pressure. Those women over thirty-five who did not smoke or have these other risk factors were not at higher risk than women under thirty-five if they used birth control pills.[8]

The birth control pills of the 1960s also had much higher doses of estrogen than that found in today's low-dose pills. We now know that lower doses of estrogen are associated with a lower risk of blood clotting problems. Thus, these newer pills are even safer than those used in the past. Still, there is this reluctance among physicians and older women to use oral contraceptives because of concerns about these possible risks.

How Does the Use of Birth Control Pills Affect Problems Such as Heart Attack and Stroke?

Concerns have been raised about birth controll pills and their effects on heart attack, stroke, venous thromboembolism (blood clots in the veins), breast cancer, fibroids, and weight.

Heart Attack

It appears that the risk of having a heart attack while on birth control pills is related mainly to other risk factors for heart disease. The most important of these are smoking, high blood pressure, and diabetes. This risk also increases with age. A healthy, nonsmoking woman over the age of thirty-five has a low risk for a heart attack. Low-dose birth control pills (which contain 35 micrograms or less of ethinyl estradiol, the estrogen in most pills) have minimal or no effect on that risk.[9] For women older than 35 who smoke, have high blood pressure, or diabetes, other options should be considered.

Stroke

The risk of stroke from birth control pills also seems to be related to other risk factors. Women who smoke, have high blood pressure, or experience migraine headaches have a higher risk of stroke when on birth control pills. Once again, healthy, nonsmoking women over the age of thirty-five have a low risk for stroke. For these women, low-dose birth control pills have a minimal effect on that risk.

Venous Thromboembolism

Venous thromboembolism is the medical term for blood clots that usually form in the deep veins of the legs or pelvis. Parts of the blood clot may break off and go to other parts of the body. This is called an embolism. When the blood clot goes to the lungs, it can block off part of the blood supply to the lung, and if enough of the blood supply is cut off, it can lead to death.

Birth control pills, even the low-dose pills, do increase the risk of venous thromboembolism. Smoking does not increase this risk. It is estimated that for every ten thousand women taking birth control pills, one to three women a year would have this problem.[10] Overall, even though there is an increase in the risk of venous thromboembolism, it is still very uncommon. Women who have certain inherited blood clotting problems may have a higher risk.

Breast Cancer

Because hormones have been implicated in breast cancer, there has been a concern that the use of birth control pills may increase its risk. Studies in the past have shown a possible connection between birth control pill use and breast cancer, but more recent studies do not show a correlation between the two.[11] If birth control pills do increase the risk, it seems to be only a very small increase.

Several large studies have shown that the combination birth control pill reduces the risk of ovarian and endometrial (lining of the uterus) cancers. Using the pill may decrease the risk of these cancers by 50 percent or more.[12] So the pill provides significant protection against the two most common gynecologic cancers in women.

Fibroids

In the past, there was a concern that birth control pills may stimulate fibroids to grow. However, the current low-dose pills do not stimulate fibroid growth and appear safe to take if fibroids are present.[13]

Weight

There is a perception that birth control pills cause weight gain. Studies of low-dose pills have not shown any significant weight gain with these products.[14] Perhaps some of the perception of weight gain was from the bloating that birth control pills can cause. However, though birth control pills do not seem to cause weight gain in women in general, individual women taking these pills may actually have problems with weight gain, and some may have problems with fluid retention, which causes weight gain. When they stop the birth control pills, their weight returns to normal.

There is some evidence that combination birth control pills are less effective in heavier women. One study showed that women who were in the top quarter in weight (over 155 pounds) had a 60 percent higher chance of getting pregnant while on the birth control pill than women under that weight.[15]

Though this sounds problematic, birth control pills are still very effective in heavier women. If you look at the chart at the effectiveness of the combination pills, the rate varies from 0.1 to 3.0 percent. A 60 percent increase would mean the pill would still be 0.16 to 4.8 percent effective, which is still much better than many other contraceptive choices. So even though birth control pills may be less effective in heavier women, they are still a very reasonable choice.

So overall, in healthy women over thirty-five, birth control pills are relatively safe.

What Are the Benefits of Birth Control Pills?

The benefits of birth control pills:

- Effectively prevent pregnancy
- Regulate menstrual cycles (even during perimenopause)
- Decrease the amount of bleeding during menstruation
- Decrease menstrual cramping
- Offer some protection from pelvic infections
- Decrease the risk of uterine and ovarian cancer
- Help to clear acne
- Reduce ovulatory pain
- Reduce ovarian cyst formation
- Improve bone density
- Decrease hot flashes, night sweats, and other perimenopausal symptoms

What Are the Disadvantages of Birth Control Pills?

The disadvantages of birth control pills:

- Possible side effects, including:
    - Nausea (taking the pill at bedtime can help prevent this)
    - Headaches
    - Breast tenderness
    - Breakthrough bleeding (spotting between periods)
    - Acne (usually it gets better, but sometimes it gets worse)
    - Decreased sex drive
    - Moodiness and irritability
    - Depression
    - Weight gain (in a small number of women)
    - Fluid retention and swelling
    - Bloating
- Only available by prescription
- Expensive
- Have to take it consistently
- May increase cholesterol
- Possible decreased effectiveness in preventing pregnancy if taking certain medications such as antiseizure medicines
- May be less effective in preventing pregnancy in heavier women

Who Shouldn't Take Birth Control Pills?

Women with any of the following should *not* take the combined pill:[16]

- Thrombophlebitis or thromboembolic disorder, or a history of them
- Stroke or a history of stroke
- Heart disease, such as coronary artery disease, heart attack, angina
- Severe liver problems
- Hepatitis
- Known or suspected breast cancer, or a history of breast cancer
- Pregnancy
- Abnormal vaginal bleeding that has not been evaluated
- Smokers older than thirty-five

Women with the following have a higher risk of problems when taking birth control pills and need to weigh the pros and cons carefully before taking the pill:[17]

- *Migraine headaches.* This may increase the risk of strokes. However, some women may have an improvement of their migraines on the pill.
- *High blood pressure.* This may increase the risk of heart attack and stroke while on the pill, but if the blood pressure is under good control, the risk is minimal in women under thirty-five.
- *Epilepsy.* Birth control pills do not worsen seizures. However, anti-seizure medications can decrease the effectiveness of the pill in preventing pregnancy.
- *Diabetes.* This may increase the risk of heart attack and stroke while on the pill, but if the diabetes is under good control, the risk is minimal in women under thirty-five.
- *Gallbladder disease.* The birth control pill may worsen symptoms if a woman already has gallstones.
- *Sickle cell disease or sickle C disease.* Birth control pills may increase the risk of thrombosis (clotting) in these women.
- *Elective surgery.* Birth control pills increase the risk of venous thrombosis (clots in the veins). Surgery of any kind also increases this risk, especially longer surgeries. Ideally, birth control pills would be discontinued four weeks before the surgery to minimize this risk. There is also some concern that being immobilized for long periods of time (even sitting on long flights) may increase the risk of venous thrombosis.
- *Breastfeeding.* The combination birth control pills that contain estrogen and progestin may decrease breast milk production. Most women who are nursing usually will be given progestin-only birth control pills, which do not affect the breast milk supply.

Perimenopause and the Pill

So what's a perimenopausal woman to do about birth control pills? For most healthy perimenopausal women, the birth control pill is a reasonable option with several other benefits that are especially pertinent to women at this stage of life, including: decreasing bleeding problems such as irregular or heavy periods; helping with hot flashes, vaginal dryness, and other symptoms of perimenopause; helping to protect the bones; and decreasing ovarian and endometrial cancer.

Which Pill Should You Use?

If you do decide to go with the pill, which one should you pick? The low-dose combination birth control pills all have the same estrogen called ethinyl estradiol. Each pill contains from 20 to 35 micrograms of ethinyl estradiol. The benefit of using less estrogen is that certain side effects such as nausea may be lessened. However, there tends to be more breakthrough bleeding (spotting between your periods) with less estrogen.

The main difference between pills is the progestin used. Progestins are synthetic compounds that act like progesterone (the hormone that helps maintain your menstrual cycle) in the body. Since every woman is different, it cannot be determined ahead of time how each woman will respond to a given estrogen and progestin combination. So finding a birth control pill that is right for you is essentially one of trial and error.

Some women can take virtually any pill without any problem, while others can take only a certain one or may not tolerate any. If you do start using birth control pills, try to continue with a given pill for three cycles before giving up on it since it can take a while for your body to get used to being on the pill.

CONTRACEPTIVE RING, PATCH, AND LUNELLE

There are three relatively new contraceptive options on the market. All three use estrogen and progestins and work basically the same way as the combination birth control pill. They have generally the same risks, benefits, and side effects as the combination birth control pill. The main difference is in how they deliver the hormones and how often they have to be given. Their main advantage lies in not having to remember to take a pill every day. This helps to decrease the likelihood of an unplanned pregnancy due to a skipped pill.

- *Nuva-Ring.* This is a silicone ring with estrogen and a progestin that is placed in the vagina. The hormones are absorbed through the vagina. The ring is inserted in the vagina and left for three weeks. It is removed for one week, during which time you have a period, and then is replaced. Some women are uncomfortable about placing the ring in their vagina or may have some discomfort when it is inside.
- *Ortho-Evra.* This is a contraceptive patch containing estrogen and a

progestin in a patch that is placed on the skin. The hormones are absorbed through the skin. The patch is replaced every week for three weeks and left off for a week during which you have a period. Breast tenderness seems to be worse when the patch is first started, but that improves over several months. It may cause skin irritation at the site of the patch. It also may be less effective in women over 198 pounds.[18]

- *Lunelle.* This is a contraceptive injection containing both estrogen and a progestin. The injection is given once a month.

These are overall good choices for women who have difficulty remembering to take a pill consistently. They are also good choices for women who travel a lot or work late shifts and have difficulty taking the pill at the same time every day (when traveling, the changes in time zones and a hectic schedule can make it difficult to be consistent with pill taking).

THE MINIPILL (PROGESTIN-ONLY PILL)

There is another birth control pill that contains only progestins (synthetic progesterone). This pill must be taken at the same time every day. A pill containing hormones is taken every day, unlike the combination birth control pill that is taken for three weeks and then skipped for a week in order for you to have your period. The minipill contains no estrogen, so it may be a good alternative for those perimenopausal women for whom estrogen-containing pills are not recommended.

Because of the very low dose of progestins, about 40 percent of women on the minipill will ovulate normally. This pill, unlike the combination pill, relies more on its effect on the cervical mucus and endometrial lining to prevent pregnancy. The progestins makes the cervical mucus thick and hard for the sperm to penetrate. They also make the endometrial lining (the lining of the uterus) unreceptive to implantation. The low-dose nature of the pill also makes it more susceptible to failure if not taken consistently. If the pill is taken more than three hours late, a back-up method is needed.

However, the low-dose nature of the minipill also makes it a good choice for certain women:

- Women who are breastfeeding. The progestin-only pill does not interfere with the production of breast milk. Ovulation is already suppressed in breastfeeding women, so this factor in combination with the minipill make for very effective contraception.

- Women over forty. The significant decrease in fertility after forty adds to the effectiveness of the minipill.
- Women who experience significant side effects from combination birth control pills. If women have severe problems with diminished libido, nausea, breast tenderness, headaches, or other side effects on the combination birth control pill, the minipill may be a good alternative.
- Women with contraindication to estrogen. Women who have cardiovascular disease, history of thromboembolism, severe diabetes, and smokers over thirty-five who are at higher risk of heart attack, stroke, and venous thromboembolism (blood clots in the veins) may choose to take the minipill. Estrogen appears to be the main culprit in increasing the risks of these problems when on the combination birth control pill. Taking the minipill may decrease the likelihood of these risks though no large scale studies have been done to prove this.

Possible downsides to the minipill include:

- It must be taken consistently. If a pill is taken more than three hours late, a back-up method is needed for the next forty-eight hours.
- It can cause irregular bleeding. The minipill can have variable effects on ovulation, which range from no changes in the cycle to shorter or longer cycles to no bleeding at all.
- It can increase acne.
- Its effectiveness is decreased when taking certain medications such as antiseizure medicines

Overall, the minipill is an effective choice for motivated women who are unable to tolerate combination birth control pills or have other medical problems as listed above.

MORNING-AFTER PILL (EMERGENCY CONTRACEPTION)

Sometimes, after an unexpected night of unprotected passion, a woman realizes she may get pregnant. This fear is not restricted to teenagers, but to all women of reproductive age. Emergency contraception is designed to be used in certain situations and should not be used routinely to prevent pregnancy. Emergency contraception can be used when condoms break, after unprotected intercourse (whether forced or consensual), or if the diaphragm or cervical cap is dislodged.

The morning-after pill needs to be taken as soon as possible after unprotected intercourse, but can be taken up to seventy-two hours afterward. The first dose is taken as soon as possible and the second dose of the same type of pill is taken twelve hours later. There are two morning-after pills currently marketed: Plan B and Preven. Plan B contains high doses of progestin, while Preven is made up of high doses of estrogen and progestin.

The morning-after pill seems to work by preventing implantation. This method fails to prevent pregnancy about 2 percent of the time. Because of the high doses of hormones in these pills, a number of side effects have been noted, including nausea, vomiting, headaches, and breast tenderness. You may need to take some other medicine for the nausea. You may also have some bleeding several days after taking these pills. If the bleeding gets very heavy, where you are soaking through a tampon in less than an hour, or if the bleeding persists for longer than a week, call your physician.

There is also some concern that the high doses of hormones could harm the fetus if the morning-after pill fails. Moreover, Preven should not be used in women who cannot take estrogen (see birth control pills).

If you rely only on condoms for contraception, you may want to keep the morning-after pill handy in case a condom breaks. It may be difficult to get on the weekend or if you're traveling. A prescription from your physician is needed to get the morning-after pill.

DEPO-PROVERA

Depo-Provera is a hormonal form of birth control that is given by injection every three months. It contains medroxyprogesterone acetate, a progestin (a synthetic hormone that acts similarly to progesterone in the body). Depo-Provera is another very effective contraceptive option for those perimenopausal women who can't use any contraception that contains estrogen.

Depo-Provera makes the cervical mucus too thick and hard for the sperm to penetrate. It also renders the endometrial lining (the lining of the uterus) unreceptive to implantation. These are the ways the minipill, described earlier, works. But the progestin level is high enough to also suppress ovulation, making this a very effective form of birth control.

Because Depo-Provera does not contain estrogen, it doesn't have many of the side effects and risks of the combination birth control pills. No increase in thrombosis (formation of blood clots) has been noted with Depo-Provera. This allows it to be considered for use in women with cardiovascular disease, history of thromboembolism, severe diabetes, smokers over thirty-five, and other women who are at higher risk of heart attack, stroke, and venous thromboembolism such as those with sickle-cell disease.

The advantages of Depo-Provera:

- Improved compliance (you only have to remember to come in once every three months for a shot)
- Very effective at preventing pregnancy
- Decreases bleeding and cramping
- Does not decrease breast milk production
- Can be used in women in whom estrogen is contraindicated
- Raises the seizure threshold (decreases the likelihood a woman with a seizure disorder will have a seizure)
- Not affected by antiseizure medications
- Decreases the risk of endometrial cancer
- May help improve symptoms from endometriosis
- May decrease sickle-cell crisis episodes

The downsides of Depo-Provera:

- Irregular bleeding
- Weight gain
- Depression and mood changes
- Breast tenderness
- Taken through injection, necessitating a visit to the physician's office every three months
- Delayed return of fertility
- If there are side effects, you have to wait over three months until the injection wears off for the side effects to disappear

Irregular bleeding is seen in 70 percent of women in the first year.[19] The bleeding is usually light. After the first year, only 10 percent of women continue to have irregular bleeding.

When the Depo-Provera is discontinued, 50 percent of women taking it will return to their normal menstrual bleeding within six months. For 25 percent of women it can take a year before they resume their normal periods.[20] Because of this, Depo-Provera users may have a delay in their fertility for up to a year after their last injection. Women who want to become pregnant should consider discontinuing the Depo-Provera a year before they wish to conceive and use a different form of birth control until they are ready to conceive.

Women with the following concerns have a higher risk of problems when taking Depo-Provera and need to weigh the pros and cons carefully before taking it:[21]

- Breast cancer
- Liver disease
- Severe heart disease
- Severe depression
- Difficulty with injections
- Desire to have a rapid return of fertility after stopping birth control

NORPLANT

The Norplant system consisted of six silastic capsules containing a progestin called levonorgestrel. The six capsules were implanted under the skin of the arm. The progestin was slowly released and prevented pregnancy for five years. At this time, it has been taken off the market.

IUD (INTRAUTERINE DEVICE)

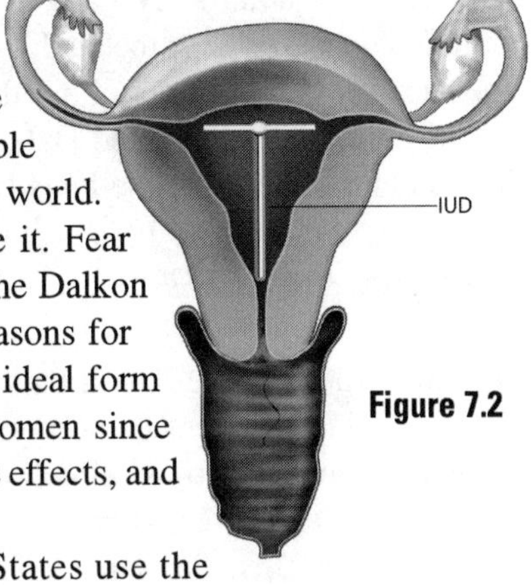

The intrauterine device or IUD is the most widely used method of reversible (nonpermanent) birth control in the world. American women, however, hardly use it. Fear of pelvic infection and problems with the Dalkon Shield IUD in the past are the main reasons for its lack of use. The IUD is actually an ideal form of contraception for perimenopausal women since it is very effective, has no hormonal side effects, and is long acting.

IUD

Figure 7.2

Since few women in the United States use the IUD, they don't have friends or family to tell them about their experience with the IUD. Many women depend on friends and family for information and advice. Fear of the unknown keeps many women from trying this effective form of birth control: "I don't want to have something inside of me."

The IUD is composed of a part that is placed in the uterus and a "tail" of thread that comes through the cervical canal into the vagina. The thread allows the user to feel that the IUD is still in place. It is also grasped and used to pull out the IUD when it is no longer needed.

Why Are So Few IUDs Used in This Country?

The modern IUD was developed during the twentieth century. A number of IUDs became available during the 1960s and 1970s. One IUD, the Dalkon Shield, was defective and associated with a high number of pelvic infections. The "tail" of thread used was multifilamented, like sewing thread, and encased in a plastic sheath. This allowed bacteria to climb from the vagina into the uterus, causing pelvic infections. The large numbers of women who developed pelvic infections led to many many lawsuits against the Dalkon Shield manufacturer, and ultimately to its bankruptcy.

Unfortunately, the negative publicity over the Dalkon Shield adversely affected all IUDs. Women feared that the IUD would lead to pelvic infection, which could potentially cause infertility. A number of other companies discontinued selling and marketing IUDs because of the cost of defending lawsuits, even though they won most of the cases.

IUDs are still available, but because of the lingering concerns about the IUD, it is not commonly used in the United States. Current IUDs use a monofilament string for the "tail," similar to fishing line. This type of string does not allow bacteria to climb the string and get into the uterus, as they did with the multifilamented Dalkon Shield string. Let's look closer at the IUD and try to separate the fears from the facts.

How Does the IUD Work?

One concern about the IUD is the way it works. Some people think that the IUD essentially causes an abortion. However, the main way IUDs seem to prevent pregnancy is by killing the sperm before it gets to the egg. The IUD in the uterus creates inflammation, which is enough to kill the sperm.[22] If fertilization occurs, the same inflammation prevents implantation. Similarly, birth control pills, Depo-Provera, the minipill, the contraceptive ring, the patch, and injection all potentially prevent implantation, thus preventing pregnancy, though that is not the primary way they work.

The IUD is inserted during an office visit. A speculum is placed in the vagina (as when a Pap smear is done). The cervix is cleaned with betadine, an iodine solution. The cervix is then grasped with an instrument and the IUD is pushed through the cervical canal into the uterus. The strings are trimmed. Sometimes an ultrasound is done after the IUD placement to ensure that it is in the correct place.

After the IUD is inserted, you should feel for the strings after each period to make sure the IUD is still there. If the strings can't be felt, or if they feel longer than normal, it could mean that the IUD has been expelled, partially expelled, or is in the wrong location. Should this occur, see your physician as soon as possible and use a backup method of birth control in the interim. If there is any unusual pain, discharge, or bleeding your physician should be notified immediately as this could be a sign of infection.

Types of IUDs

There are two types of IUDs. One contains copper while the other contains progestins. The copper IUD is good for ten years while the progestin IUD (Mirena) is good for five. The main advantage of the progestin IUD is that you tend to have lighter periods than with the copper IUD. The main disadvantages are that some women have irregular bleeding or no bleeding at all and it lasts half as long as the copper IUD.

The benefits of IUDs:

- Very reliable
- Good long-term contraception (the copper IUD is good for ten years, the Mirena is good for five years)
- No hormonal side effects (with the copper IUD)
- Does not decrease breast milk production
- Can be used in women in whom estrogen is contraindicated
- Prompt return of fertility after removal

The downsides of IUDs:

- Heavier menstrual bleeding with the copper IUD (the progestin containing IUD usually decreases bleeding over time)

- Increased cramping (with the copper IUD, cramping is usually the worst for several months after placement of the IUD; less cramping is seen with the progestin-containing IUD)
- Discomfort during the insertion
- Small increased risk of pelvic infection in the month after insertion
- Increased risk of pelvic infection if exposed to sexually transmitted diseases
- No protection from sexually transmitted diseases
- Partner may feel the strings during intercourse
- Generally recommended for women in a mutually monogamous relationship who have already had children

Some women don't like the idea of having something inside their body. However, for many women, especially after they have had several children and are in a stable, long-term relationship, this can be an ideal form of birth control without any of the hormonal side effects seen with the birth control pill or Depo-provera.

STERILIZATION

Tubal Ligation versus Vasectomy

Sterilization is the most common form of contraception used in perimenopausal women. Sterilization can be done on either men or women, and both are effective forms of birth control. However, both should be considered permanent and irreversible. Which is right for you and your partner?

Generally, vasectomy is a safer and simpler procedure than tubal ligation. Vasectomy is done with local anesthesia: The physician injects lidocaine or another local anesthetic to numb the area. Tubal ligation is usually done under general anesthesia. With general anesthesia, you are put to sleep, your body is paralyzed, and a machine breathes for you. General anesthesia, though usually safe, is still significantly more risky than local anesthesia.

A vasectomy is performed in the physician's office. Only two tiny cuts are needed to find the vas deferens, the tube that carries the sperm from the testicle (where it is made) to the urethra (where it is expelled). The vas deferens is cut and tied. No vital structures are near the vas deferens that can be damaged (though your partner may disagree).

Tubal ligation is performed in the operating room. A cut is made in the

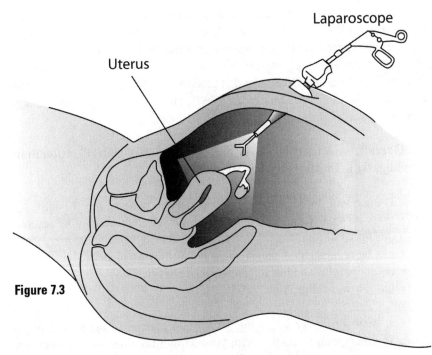

Figure 7.3

belly button and the laparoscope is placed through the opening into your belly. Your bowels, bladder, and major blood vessels lie near the fallopian tubes and can in rare cases be injured during the surgery to block your fallopian tubes. In *very* rare cases, this can be fatal. Under any circumstances, there is generally more pain and a longer recovery after tubal ligation than vasectomy (see below for more on tubal ligation and the procedure).

After the vasectomy, a sperm count is done to confirm that the surgery successfully blocked the vas deferens. A backup method should be used until no more sperm are seen. After a tubal ligation, there is no testing to see if the tubes are blocked. You will know if it didn't work only if you become pregnant.

Sterilization Can Fail

Both vasectomy and tubal ligation can fail. The tubes in both men and women can grow back together (the body tries to fix what is damaged, even when it is done purposely), leading to possible future pregnancy. The failure rate for tubal ligation is about 1 in 300, while the failure rate for vasectomy is about 1 in 1000.[23] If a vasectomy fails, the result is pregnancy. If a tubal ligation fails, the woman has a much higher chance of a tubal pregnancy, which may be life threatening if not detected and treated in time.

A study several years ago revealed that men who had had a vasectomy were at higher risk of getting prostate cancer. Other researchers looking at this study and studies since have disputed this correlation.[24] However, this association is still occasionally used by men to avoid vasectomy (many men will try almost any excuse to avoid being cut).

Overall, vasectomy is a safer and simpler form of sterilization than tubal ligation. To summarize, vasectomy:

- is done with local anesthesia as opposed to general anesthesia;
- risks no vital structures such as the bowels, which may be injured during tubal ligation;
- can be tested with a sperm count to confirm its success;
- is less painful and has a shorter recovery time; and
- has a lower failure rate.

The main difficulty is getting your male partner to agree to have it done. You may want to discuss with your partner the pros and cons of each procedure, emphasizing the fact that vasectomy is easier, cheaper, and has a much lower risk of serious complications than a tubal ligation. You could always say, "Hey, I carried the pregnancies and gave birth to the kids, now it's *your* turn to have the vasectomy." Then let him choose. You could always offer abstinence as an alternative. After all, abstinence is the most effective form of birth control.

Tubal Ligation

Tubal ligation is a surgical procedure done in the operating room. It can be done at the time of a cesarean section, after a vaginal delivery, or at any other time by laparoscopy. The purpose of a tubal ligation is to block the fallopian tubes so that the egg and sperm cannot meet, thus preventing pregnancy.

Laparoscopic tubal ligation is usually done as outpatient surgery. After you have made the decision to be permanently sterilized and are completely sure that you don't want any more children (and your partner will not agree to a vasectomy), you may schedule this procedure with a gynecologic surgeon.

Ideally, a tubal ligation is done during the first half of your cycle before you ovulate. If it is done after you have ovulated, there is a small chance that the egg may have been fertilized but it may still be too early to detect it on a blood pregnancy test. That could lead to your having surgery when you are unknowingly pregnant, thus potentially exposing the fetus to many possibly harmful medications.

You will probably want to take one to two weeks off from work to recover from the surgery. Ideally, you will have someone to help around the house for a day or two after surgery.

The Procedure

At your pre-op meeting with the surgeon, he or she will describe the procedure, the alternatives, risks, and benefits. He or she will answer any questions you may have.

Once you are put to sleep in the operating room through anesthesia, your bladder is usually drained with a catheter (a small tube). (Your bladder is drained to keep it out of the way during the surgery.) The catheter may make your urethra (the opening to your bladder) sore or irritated after surgery. The irritation should subside within one to two days. If it does not, or if it worsens, it could mean that you have a bladder infection and may need to be treated. Bring it to the attention of your surgeon if you have this problem.

After your bladder is drained, your abdomen is filled with carbon dioxide gas in order to see the organs clearly. Carbon dioxide can be irritating to the diaphragm (the muscle at the base of your lungs that makes you breathe). When you wake up, the irritation of the diaphragm is felt in your shoulder blades. At the end of the surgery, as much of the gas is removed as possible, but some stays behind. This gas takes several days to be reabsorbed by your body and it is during this time that you feel most of the pain in your shoulder blades.

The laparoscope is a long tube through which the surgeon can see into your body. The laparoscope is placed through an incision in your belly button into your abdomen. Another small incision may be made a couple inches above your pubic bone to put other instruments into your abdomen to perform the tubal ligation.

Laparoscopic tubal ligation can be done in several ways. The way it is done depends on the preference of your surgeon. There is no great advantage of one procedure over another.

The warning signs of complications include:

- Fever or chills (which could be a sign of infection)
- Worsening pain
- Redness around the cut
- Pus draining from the cut

You need to call your surgeon immediately if you experience any of these problems.

Essure

The newest method of sterilization is called Essure. A tiny coil embedded with a mesh is placed through the vagina into the uterus with a hystero-scope into each fallopian tube. The coils irritate the lining of the tube, causing scar tissue to form, thus blocking the tubes. It can take three months for the scar tissue to block the tube completely, so a backup meth-od of contraception has to be used during that time. After three months, an X-ray test is done to make sure the tubes are blocked.

Essure is still new to the United States and its long-term effectiveness is still being determined.

PREGNANCY

For those women who become pregnant out of choice or by chance, this can be a time of anxiety and concern. Most women are aware that after forty there is an increased risk of having a baby with Down's syndrome. There are a number of other potential problems that increase as the mother ages. Fortunately, most pregnancies end happily with a healthy mother and baby.

In women over age forty, the following risks are increased:[25]

- Infant with Down's syndrome or other chromosomal abnormalities
- Miscarriage
- Gestational diabetes (diabetes during pregnancy)
- Hypertensive disorders of pregnancy
- Stillbirth
- Need for cesarean section

Gestational diabetes and hypertensive disorders may be related to obesity, which is more common in older women. Studies have shown that when obesity was factored out, the increase in these risks disappeared.[26] The increase in risk for cesarean section seems to be related to the aging uterus not contracting as effectively. The other risks such as chromosomal abnormalities, miscarriage, and stillbirth are more directly related to age.

Genetic Testing

Genetic testing will generally be offered to women thirty-five and older because of their increased risk of having a baby with a chromosomal abnormality. Normally, there are twenty-three pairs of chromosomes. Down's syndrome, where there is an extra twenty-first chromosome, is the most common chromosomal abnormality known. Other chromosomal problems include extra or missing parts of chromosomes, which usually result in miscarriage, stillbirth, or severe developmental problems if the baby survives.

Two main types of testing are offered: chorionic villus sampling and amniocentesis. Chorionic villus sampling is done at the end of the first trimester (the first third of the pregnancy), around the eleventh and twelfth weeks of pregnancy. A needle is placed through the vagina and some of the placental tissue is sampled and sent to the lab to be cultured. After one to two weeks when enough cells have grown, the chromosomes are analyzed and actually counted. If there is an extra twenty-first chromosome, the baby has Down's syndrome. Other chromosomal problems can also be discovered this way.

Amniocentesis is usually done around fifteen to seventeen weeks into the pregnancy. A needle is placed through your abdomen into the uterus to collect some of the fluid surrounding the baby. The fluid contains cells from the baby, which are then grown in the lab. The chromosomes are analyzed and counted as described above. The same information can be obtained.

The main advantage of chorionic villus sampling is that it can be done earlier than amniocentesis. If there is a problem with the baby and the mother chooses to abort, it is easier and safer earlier in the pregnancy. However, the risk of miscarriage is higher as a result of chorionic villus sampling than after amniocentesis. With either test, the cells may not grow and the test may be inconclusive, or the test may be contaminated with the mother's cells, giving a false normal result. Amniocentesis is slightly more reliable than chorionic villus sampling.

Blood tests are also available and may show if you have a higher chance of having a baby with Down's syndrome or other chromosomal abnormalities, but they still miss a significant percentage of cases. The test can also falsely show a higher risk, though the baby may be normal. This leads to anxiety and further testing such as an amniocentesis to determine that all is normal. Ultrasound has also been able to pick up a number of fetuses with chromosomal abnormalities, but also misses a significant number.

Nevertheless, the prognosis is good in the majority of pregnancies of women over thirty-five, especially for healthy women of normal weight. The best advice for women contemplating pregnancy is to maintain a healthy weight, stay active, eat healthy, and take prenatal vitamins. Prenatal vitamins should be started two months before trying to conceive in order to get folate levels up. This helps decrease the chance of neural tube defects, a birth defect in which there is an opening over the baby's spinal cord or brain.

THE BOTTOM LINE

Women during perimenopause need contraception. The high percentages of unplanned pregnancies in women at this time attest to this. Unless you want to have children, you need to look into the many contraceptive alternatives available to you. Even if you don't need contraception because of tubal ligation or hysterectomy, condom use is still beneficial in preventing certain sexually transmitted infections if you start a new relationship. And if you do want to get pregnant, even though it may be harder to get pregnant and there are more risks associated with pregnancy at this time, most pregnancies end well for both mother and baby.

CHAPTER 8

SINGLE AGAIN AND AVOIDING SEXUALLY TRANSMITTED DISEASES

*S*ingle again. Many of you may now find yourself in a situation that you never expected. Whether you are divorced, separated, or widowed, you are now single after having been one half of a pair. Starting a new relationship can be exciting and even exhilarating if you meet someone who clicks with you. However, dating brings up issues that you may not have had to deal with for many years, such as birth control and possible exposure to sexually transmitted diseases.

Birth control may or may not be an issue for you. However, if your ex had a vasectomy, you may now have to think about birth control again. (Chapter 7 reviews the pros and cons of the different birth control options.)

Sexually transmitted diseases are another unpleasant but important concern. There are several sexually transmitted infections that you have to worry about:

- Chlamydia
- Gonorrhea
- Herpes
- HIV
- Hepatitis A, B, and C
- Trichomonas
- Human papillomavirus

- Syphilis
- Molluscum contagiosum
- Pubic lice
- Lymphogranuloma venereum
- Chancroid
- And other rare diseases

Unfortunately, sexually transmitted diseases are more likely to be spread from man to woman than woman to man, and women tend to have more serious long-term consequences from sexually transmitted diseases. We will discuss the more common sexually transmitted diseases in more detail below. The following table gives you an idea of how common certain sexually transmitted infections are.

Common Sexually Transmitted Diseases[1]

STD	Incidence Nationally (Estimated Number of New Cases each Year)	Prevalence Nationally (Estimated Number of People Currently Infected)*
Chlamydia	3 million	2 million
Gonorrhea	650,000	Not available
Herpes	1 million	45 million
Human Papillomavirus (HPV)	5.5 million	20 million
Syphilis	70,000	Not available
Hepatitis B	120,000	417,000
Trichomoniasis	5 million	Not available
Human immunodeficiency virus	40,000	338,000 (MMWR 2000)

*No recent surveys on national prevalence for gonorrhea, syphilis, or trichomoniasis have been conducted.

CHLAMYDIA

Chlamydia is a sexually transmitted disease caused by a bacteria called *Chlamydia trachomatis*. About three million Americans are infected with chlamydia every year.[2] Chlamydia can be spread by vaginal, anal, or oral sex. Unfortunately, three quarters of infected women and half of infected men have no symptoms, making it difficult to discover.

Symptoms

The chlamydia bacteria spreads from the man's penis and can infect the cervix, urethra (the opening of the bladder), rectum, or throat, depending on the type of sex you have. When the cervix or urethra is infected, you may experience an abnormal vaginal discharge or burning during urination. The infection can spread to the fallopian tubes and can cause pelvic or low back pain, pain with intercourse, fever, nausea, and abnormal bleeding.

Chlamydia infection in the rectum or throat may cause rectal pain or sore throat. Men can have a discharge from their penis, burning with urination, or pain and swelling in the testicles. If you have symptoms, they usually show up one to three weeks after exposure.

Complications

Chlamydia can result in long-term problems, even if you have no symptoms. The infection can cause scarring in the Fallopian tubes, leading to infertility, ectopic pregnancy, and chronic pelvic pain. An ectopic pregnancy is a life-threatening condition to the mother where the pregnancy grows outside of the uterus, usually in the Fallopian tube. If the pregnancy is in the Fallopian tube, it can grow to the point where it ruptures the tube, causing severe bleeding in the mother and potentially death.

Chlamydia may increase your risk of being infected with HIV if you are exposed to the virus. Chlamydia can be passed to a baby as he or she goes through the birth canal, causing an eye infection or pneumonia.

Diagnosis

Chlamydia can be detected by collecting a specimen from the cervix. A newer test can detect chlamydia in the urine. Chlamydia can also be diagnosed by testing the rectum or throat if those areas are infected.

Treatment

Antibiotics are used to treat chlamydia. Your partner(s) should also be treated.

Prevention

Your best protection against chlamydia when you are dating is to have any partner tested *before* you have intercourse and to use condoms every time you have intercourse.

GONORRHEA

Gonorrhea is an infection caused by the bacteria *Neisseria gonorrhoeae*. About 650,000 Americans are infected with gonorrhea each year.[3] Gonorrhea can be spread by vaginal, anal, or oral sex. Many women have mild or no symptoms of infection but the majority of men have symptoms including a discharge from the penis, burning during urination, and painful or swollen testicles.

Symptoms

Gonorrhea can infect the cervix, urethra, rectum, or throat, depending on the type of sex you have. Symptoms usually occur in three to five days. When the cervix or urethra is infected, you may have an abnormal vaginal discharge or bleeding or burning with urination. When the infection spreads to the fallopian tubes, it can cause pelvic or lower back pain, pain with intercourse, fever, nausea, and abnormal bleeding. Infection of the rectum can cause discharge, pain, itching, and bleeding.

Complications

Gonorrhea can cause scarring in the Fallopian tubes, leading to infertility, ectopic pregnancy (pregnancy outside of the uterus), and chronic pelvic pain. Gonorrhea can infect the blood or joints, causing a life-threatening infection. Having gonorrhea can increase your risk of getting HIV if you are exposed to this virus. Even if you have no symptoms, you may have these long-term problems. Gonorrhea can be passed to a baby as he or she goes through the birth canal, causing a serious infection or blindness.

It is estimated that a man has a 20 to 25 percent chance of becoming infected with gonorrhea during a single sexual encounter with an infected woman. However, a woman has about an 80 to 90 percent chance of becoming infected during a single sexual encounter with an infected man.[4] Life is not fair!

Diagnosis

Gonorrhea can be diagnosed by collecting a specimen from the cervix or the urine. It can also be picked up by testing the rectum or throat if those areas are infected.

Treatment

Antibiotics are used to treat gonorrhea. Your partner(s) should also be treated.

Prevention

Your best protection against gonorrhea is to have any partner tested before you have intercourse and to use condoms every time you have intercourse.

HERPES

Herpes is an infection caused by herpes simplex viruses type 1(HSV-1) and type 2 (HSV-2). Each year, one million more people are infected with genital herpes. Since you can never get rid of this virus, a total of forty-five million people, or one out of five adults, is infected with genital herpes in the United States.[5] More women than men are infected with HSV-2, probably due to the fact that it is easier for a woman to become infected than men when exposed to this virus.

Symptoms

Herpes can cause painful blisters in the genital and rectal areas that break and leave very tender sores. The herpes virus can also infect other areas, such as the throat, mouth, thigh, fingers, and eyes. The first outbreak is usually the worst, lasting two to four weeks. It can also produce fever, headache, fatigue, and muscle aches.

Outbreaks may recur monthly, but are generally much less frequent. The recurrent outbreaks are almost always less severe and shorter than the first episode. Many people, nonetheless, have minimal or no symptoms when they become infected with the herpes virus. Though the herpes virus stays in your body for life, the number of outbreaks becomes less frequent with time.

You can get genital herpes by having vaginal, anal, or oral sex with someone who is infected, even if that person has no symptoms of the infection. If someone has an active herpes lesion, he or she is much more likely to pass on the infection. However, even when a person has no symptoms or sores, he or she can still be actively releasing the virus and can infect others.

If someone gets fever blisters or cold sores, which is typically caused by HSV-1, this virus can be spread to the genital area during oral sex and produce identical symptoms to genital herpes caused by HSV-2. Though HSV-1 generally causes the oral form of herpes and HSV-2 causes the genital form, they can both infect either the oral or genital area and cause similar symptoms.

Any genital-to-genital, oral-to-genital, or oral-to-oral contact can potentially pass the herpes virus, even without penetration or deep (tongue) kissing. Of course, the more contact there is, the higher the likelihood of infection. Once again, a person can pass the virus even without symptoms.

The herpes virus can also be spread from one part of your body to another by a process called autoinoculation. You could potentially spread the virus from your mouth to your genital area or vice versa by physically carrying the virus from one area to the other. If you had cold sores and were to touch your mouth when you were shedding the herpes virus and then touch your genital area, that could possibly lead to a herpes infection in the genital area.

Complications

Herpes can also be spread from a pregnant mother to her baby, usually as the baby passes through the birth canal. To prevent this, a C-section is recommended if you have an active genital herpes lesion when you are in labor. Herpes infections in newborn babies are serious and can be fatal. If you don't have an active lesion, the risk of passing the herpes virus is extremely low, so C-section is not recommended.

Herpes also makes a person more susceptible to infection by the HIV virus.

Diagnosis

Genital herpes is diagnosed through examination by a physician during an outbreak. Viral cultures and tests that detect parts of the herpes virus are normally done on an active lesion to confirm the diagnosis. *A negative test does not mean that the lesion is not herpes.* A number of factors can make the test come back negative even though herpes is there. The best time to take these tests is early in the outbreak when the virus is most plentiful.

Blood tests can also be done, but some of the older tests are not good at differentiating between HSV-1 and HSV-2. The blood test detects antibodies to HSV-1 and HSV-2. This is a problem because so many people already have antibodies to HSV-1, which means that if the test is positive you can't be sure if it is detecting HSV-1 or a new HSV-2 infection. Newer tests are better able to distinguish between HSV-1 and HSV-2. However, if a person has genital herpes caused by HSV-1, the HSV-2 test would come back negative, making that person think she doesn't have genital herpes when in fact she does. Therefore, testing the active lesion for either herpes virus is the best way to make the diagnosis.

Treatment

Medications are available that can help shorten the course of the first or recurrent outbreaks, but there is no cure for herpes. The earlier you start treatment, the better it works. Currently there are three oral medications available: acyclovir (Zovirax), valacyclovir (Valtrex), and famciclovir (Famvir). Topical antiviral ointments are also available, but are not as effective as the oral medications.

For people with frequent outbreaks (usually six or more a year), many, under a physician's supervision, are taking the medication daily to reduce the number of outbreaks. Daily therapy not only reduces the number of outbreaks, but it also decreases the amount of viral shedding that occurs without symptoms. This may reduce the risk of passing on the virus, but does not eliminate it.

Prevention

Protecting yourself against herpes is difficult. Condoms may help some, but the virus can be spread from areas not covered by the condom. Avoiding sex with someone with an active oral or genital lesion will decrease the risk of acquiring the virus, but the virus can be passed on even when there are no lesions or symptoms. And many people don't even know they carry the virus. They may never have had any significant symptoms and yet still carry the virus, unknowingly placing their sexual partners at risk. And to top it off, women are more susceptible to getting the infection than men.

So what's a woman to do? Since there is no good way to protect your-self against genital herpes, you must decide whether sex with someone is worth the risk of potentially exposing yourself to this infection. If you decide to have sex, you should still use condoms, but do so knowing that it is not a very good defense against herpes.

HUMAN PAPILLOMAVIRUS (HPV)

Human papillomavirus or HPV is a group of sexually transmitted viruses that can infect the genital area. There are over one hundred types of HPV, of which over thirty can infect the genitalia. The other types cause warts on other parts of the body. Genital HPV infections are spread mostly by sexual contact. Over 50 percent of sexually active men and women will be infected with this virus over the course of their life. An estimated 5.5 million Americans get infected every year.[6] HPV is the most common sexually transmitted infection today.

Symptoms and Complications of HPV

The biggest problem with HPV is that most people have no symptoms and don't know that they are infected. They can unknowingly pass on the virus to their partner. The problems HPV can cause in women are genital warts, cervical dysplasia, and cervical cancer. The virus gets into the cells, making them look and grow abnormally, which then causes cervical dysplasia. Certain types of HPV (including types 16, 18, 31, 33) are considered high-risk types and are more likely to cause the cervical dysplasia that progress to cervical cancer. Pap smears are used to screen for cervical changes caused by HPV.

Genital Warts

Genital warts can appear in the vagina, on the cervix, the vulva, labia, or anus. On a man, the warts can appear on the penis, scrotum, and anus. Occasionally, the warts may also be found on the thigh, the areas covered by pubic hair, and buttocks. Genital warts may take on different appearances: they may be cauliflowerlike, dome-shaped, or have a thick crustlike layer similar to common skin warts. The warts may cause some itching, burning, or bleeding, though these symptoms are rare. They usually show up within several weeks or months after becoming infected with HPV.

Genital warts can stay the same, disappear, or grow in number and size over time if left untreated. The genital warts can be treated by your placing medications on the warts or by your physician destroying them with acid or other chemicals, laser, freezing, or cutting them off. Different treatment regimens are available, but it usually takes several treatment sessions to completely destroy the warts. However, during the first six months, the genital warts are much more likely to recur, with new warts popping up even with treatment.

Abnormal Pap Smears and Cervical Dysplasia

Cervical cancer is one of the few cancers that has a preinvasive stage that is easily treatable. This stage, called cervical dysplasia, is detected by the Pap smear (this is part of the reason why Pap smears have been so successful in decreasing cervical cancer in this country). Cervical dysplasia is a condition in which the cells of the cervix have changed. It is graded as mild, moderate, or severe dysplasia according to one classification system.

Sometimes, the cervical cells are slightly abnormal in appearance. They are not abnormal enough to call dysplasia, but they are not quite normal either. A Pap smear in this gray zone is called "*a*typical *s*quamous *c*ells of *u*ndetermined *s*ignificance" or "ASCUS." Because we now know that most cervical dysplasia is caused by the human papillomavirus and what we really want to know is whether these abnormal cells are really dysplasia, many times the Pap smears that come back with ASCUS are tested for the presence of the human papillomavirus. If human papillomavirus is detected with an ASCUS Pap smear, there is a significant chance that cervical dysplasia is present and is evaluated the same way.

Cervical Cancer

HPV is now known to cause most cervical cancers. An estimated 12,900 new cases of cervical cancer were diagnosed in the United States in 2001.[7] Fortunately, this number is significantly lower than the number of cases many years ago due to by the advent of the Pap smear. (The Pap smear is a test developed by Dr. George Papanicolaou in the 1940s to screen for cervical cancer.)

The risk factors that increase the odds of cervical cancer include:

- Early onset of sexual activity
- Multiple sexual partners
- Sexual behavior of male partner
- Smoking
- Suppressed immune system

Diagnosis

Your physician diagnoses genital warts by viewing the lesions that typically appear. Sometimes a biopsy is done to confirm the diagnosis. Pap smears are used to screen for cervical dysplasia and cancer.

There are tests for HPV, but the usefulness of these tests is still being debated. The main purpose of this test is to help determine if a slightly abnormal Pap smear needs to be evaluated further. However, if someone tests positive for HPV but has no warts and no abnormal Pap smear, she will likely be told that she should still have an annual Pap smear, but not more frequently since HPV cannot be treated. Only the problems HPV causes, such as warts and cervical dysplasia, can be treated (see below). And most people who have HPV have no problems from it. Also remember that condoms won't protect your partner from HPV since the virus can be spread by skin-to-skin contact from areas that are not protected by a condom. Since nothing changes based on the results of this test, if you are not having any problems the test is not routinely done at this time.

Newer Technologies for Cervical Screening

Though the story of the Pap smear has been one of great success, it is not a perfect test. The Pap smear may miss cervical dysplasia or even cervical cancer up to 30 percent of the time.[8] However, Pap smears have still been very effective in preventing cervical cancer because it takes years, even decades, for the mild dysplasia to progress to cancer; women are therefore advised to be screened every year.[9]

New methods of improving on the venerable Pap smear have been introduced in an attempt to lower the chance of missing any abnormalities. With the traditional Pap smear, the cells are collected on a spatula and/or brush, smeared on a slide, and sprayed with a fixative. When the cells are placed on the slide, they tend to clump together and other material such as blood and mucus may make it harder to see the cells.

ThinPrep

ThinPrep is one liquid-based system where the cells are collected in the usual fashion but are then placed in a container that contains a special liquid. The container is then sent to the laboratory where a machine separates the cervical cells from other material, such a blood and mucus. The cells are then placed on a slide in a more uniform way, making it easier to evaluate the cells and detect any abnormalities.

The ThinPrep method has been shown to be more effective than the traditional Pap smear in detecting cervical dysplasia.[10] The other advantage of ThinPrep is that if the result is ASCUS, HPV testing can usually be done on the same specimen. HPV cannot be tested from the traditional Pap smear slide.

Computer Screening of Pap Smears

Computer screening of Pap smears has also been used to improve the detection rate of the Pap smear. AutoPap optically scans the slide and selects the areas most likely to represent abnormal cells. These images are then reviewed by medical personnel.[11] Currently, computer screening would probably be best used to rescreen normal Pap smears in order to detect the abnormalities missed by the cytologist. In the future as this technology improves, it may replace humans in the screening process of Pap smears.

The main disadvantage to these new technologies is cost. Liquid-based systems and computer screening both increase the cost of the Pap smear. Insurance may cover the added cost or you may have to pay for it out of pocket. You have to decide whether the added cost is worth the benefit.

How Often Do You Need a Pap Smear?

A continuing controversy in cervical cancer screening is the question of how often Pap smears should be done. The American Cancer Society and the American College of Obstetricians and Gynecologists recommend annual Pap smears for sexually active women until three adequate negative smears have been obtained. Testing after that time is at the discretion of the clinician, but continued annual testing is encouraged for women who are at higher risk for cervical cancer.

Because Pap smears can miss the abnormal cells up to 30 percent of the time, some experts recommend continued yearly Pap smears so that if there is an abnormality missed, it could be picked up a year later.[12] This is reasonable since it usually takes years or decades for the cervical cells to go from normal to mild dysplasia, to severe dysplasia, and finally to cancer.[13] Even if women choose to space their Pap smears out, breast exams, blood pressure checks, and other testing should be done on a yearly basis for most perimenopausal and menopausal women. The biggest risk factor for cervical cancer is the failure to have a Pap smear at all.

Colposcopy

If the Pap smear shows that you have cervical dysplasia or ASCUS with the human papillomavirus, you will be scheduled for a colposcopy. The Pap smear is a screening test and is good at picking up abnormal cells, but cannot tell you exactly what is happening to your cervix. A colposcopy is done to determine if the abnormalities are as bad or worse than what the Pap smear shows and how large an area is involved.

How Colposcopy Is Done

A colposcopy is a diagnostic procedure performed at your doctor's office to further evaluate your cervix after you have had an abnormal Pap smear. The first part is like a Pap smear, where a speculum is placed in your vagina to see your cervix. The colposcope is basically a microscope that gives a close-up view of the cervix so that any abnormalities can be better seen. Vinegar (acetic acid) is placed on your cervix. This may sting slightly but it helps highlight any abnormalities on your cervix so that they are easier to detect. An iodine solution called Lugol's solution may also be used to highlight any abnormal areas.

Your doctor will take a biopsy of the most abnormal-looking areas. When the biopsy is done, you will feel a sharp cramping, but it is usually over very quickly. The biopsy is sent to a lab and the results will determine what treatment you may need. Any bleeding you may have from the biopsy is controlled with the use of different substances such as silver nitrate.

You may have some spotting and discharge for several days after the colposcopy. There may be some stuff that looks like dark grains of sand mixed with your discharge. This should all clear by the end of a week. Usually, you will be told to abstain from using tampons, douching, or having vaginal intercourse for several days after the colposcopy.

Treatment

Unfortunately, the human papillomavirus itself cannot be treated. By treating genital warts or cervical dysplasia, the problems caused by HPV can be treated, but the virus itself cannot be eradicated.

Cervical dysplasia is commonly referred to as precancerous cells. Though it is true that cervical dysplasia can progress to become cervical cancer, most of the time it does not. The treatment of cervical dysplasia is evolving. Currently, if you have mild dysplasia, you can either have it treated or followed with more frequent Pap smears. Your body's immune system may get rid of the cervical dysplasia, so following it is a reasonable option.

If you have moderate or severe dysplasia, it should be treated because there is a higher likelihood that it will progress to cancer. Cervical dysplasia is treated by destroying it with laser or freezing, by removing it by a LEEP (Loop Electrosurgical Excision Procedure), or by cone biopsy. With LEEP, a wire with electricity running through it is used to remove the cervical dysplasia. LEEP is done either in the office or in outpatient surgery.

A cone biopsy is a surgical procedure done in outpatient surgery where a cone-shaped piece of the cervix containing the cervical dysplasia is excised using a scalpel or laser. After any of these procedures, more frequent Pap smears are done at four- to six-month intervals to make sure the dysplasia is gone and not recurring.

In most people, the presence of HPV is undetectable after two years of having contracted it. However, that does not mean that the virus is gone; it just isn't detectable by our current testing. Most likely, the virus persists in small amounts in the cells in the genital area. Fortunately, the immune system is generally able to keep them from causing more problems once the initial infection subsides.

Since the HPV is still present, it can still be passed to a sexual partner. Rarely, a mother can pass the virus to her baby as he or she passes through the birth canal. The virus can grow on the baby's vocal cords and cause problems, but this is very rare. A C-section is not recommended for women with genital warts or cervical dysplasia because the likelihood of passing on the HPV to the baby is so rare and the C-section poses more risks to the mother than vaginal birth.

HPV and Your Partner

If you have HPV, what does your partner need to do? He or she should probably be examined by a physician to make sure there are no genital warts. Sometimes, the warts are very small and inconspicuous, making them hard to see. If he or she has no genital warts (and for a female partner, a normal Pap smear), no further treatment is needed. Your treatment would depend on how and where the HPV manifests itself.

Now what if you've been in a mutually monogamous relationship with no other partners for many years and you are diagnosed with HPV, either manifesting as an abnormal Pap smear or genital warts? Does this mean your partner has been unfaithful? Maybe, but not necessarily. The HPV may have been dormant in you or your partner for many years and may now be manifesting clinically.

Perhaps the virus has managed to break past your immune defenses that had kept it in check for so long. An extreme example of this is in women who have had organ transplants. When they are placed on drugs that suppress their immune system in order to prevent rejection of their new transplanted organ, some of these women will then develop abnormal Pap smears or genital warts despite not having been exposed to any new sexual partners. Could something to a lesser degree happen so that the HPV surfaces in a healthy individual? It is possible. So your partner may be off the hook. But then again, he or she may not be. You will have to take other things into consideration before assuming that your partner has been unfaithful.

Prevention

Protecting yourself from HPV is difficult because the virus can be passed from areas not covered by condoms. Any genital-to-genital contact puts you at risk for becoming infected with HPV. You may think, "Hey, I've already got HPV. I don't have to worry." Not true. There are over thirty types of HPV. If you were exposed to a different HPV type, you could develop new warts or abnormal Pap smears.

Vaccines are being developed and may provide the best protection against HPV. Unfortunately, the vaccine will probably help only those who have never been exposed to HPV before.

SYPHILIS

Treponema pallidum is the bacterium that causes the sexually transmitted infection known as syphilis. About seventy thousand Americans are infected with syphilis a year.[14] Syphilis is spread through direct contact with syphilis sores, which can occur on the external genitals, in the vagina, rectum, and occasionally on the lips or in the mouth. So this infection can be spread by vaginal, anal, and oral sex. Syphilis can also be spread during later stages of the infection when the sore has healed and is no longer visible.

Symptoms

When a person is infected with syphilis, the disease goes through different stages if it is not treated. During the first stage, called the primary stage, one or more painless sores called chancres appear. These sores are seen ten to ninety days after a person becomes infected. Chancre sores look like hard round bug bites. It is where the syphilis bacteria entered the body. It lasts for three to six weeks and heals on its own.

If not treated in the first stage, the syphilis will enter the second stage, which is marked by a rash that doesn't itch. The rash can appear as the sore is fading or several weeks after the sore is gone. The rash is usually seen on the palms of the hands or the bottoms of the feet, and looks like rough red or brownish spots. The rash clears up on its own. Sometimes the rashes are so faint that they are missed. Other symptoms at this time may include fever, muscle aches, fatigue, headache, swollen lymph glands, weight loss, and patchy hair loss.

Latent syphilis, the next stage, has no symptoms. The syphilis stays hidden in the body and may start to damage the brain, nerves, eyes, heart, liver, bones, and joints. If the infection progresses, problems may emerge years later, such as blindness, loss of coordination, dementia, and death.

Syphilis in a pregnant woman can infect the baby before birth, leading to stillbirth or developmental delay, seizures, and other serious problems.

Diagnosis

Syphilis can be diagnosed by a special microscope test or more accurately by a blood test.

Treatment

Antibiotics are used to treat syphilis and should also be used to treat sexual partners. However, if the syphilis has already damaged the organs, the damage cannot be undone.

Prevention

Condoms may help somewhat against syphilis, but the infection may still be passed through areas not covered by the condom. Condoms are still useful in preventing other sexually transmitted infections and should therefore be used. Testing yourself and your potential partner before you become sexually intimate would also help provide protection against this infection and others.

HEPATITIS B

Many people don't consider hepatitis B to be a sexually transmitted infection, but it can definitely be spread by sexual contact. Hepatitis B is a virus that infects the liver and is spread through body fluids such as blood, semen, saliva, and vaginal secretions. The virus in these body fluids can enter another person's body through sex, sharing needles when using drugs, being stuck by a sharp object that has body fluids on it (working in a hospital, getting a tattoo), or giving birth (an infected mother can transfer the infection to her baby). Each year about 120,000 people become infected with hepatitis B.[15]

Symptoms

Symptoms of hepatitis B infection include jaundice (a yellow coloring of the skin and eyes caused by too much bilirubin in the blood), fatigue, loss of appetite, nausea, vomiting, and abdominal pain. The symptoms usually resolve over four to eight weeks. About 30 percent of infected people have no signs or symptoms.[16] Most people recover and develop an immunity to hepatitis B. Once the infection is cleared, that person cannot pass it on to anyone else.

However, up to 5 percent of people with hepatitis B are unable to clear the infection and become chronic carriers of this virus. This group can still pass on the hepatitis B virus to others. The infection can damage the liver and lead to cirrhosis and even death. This group of individuals are also at higher risk of developing liver cancer.[17]

Diagnosis

Hepatitis B is diagnosed by testing your blood.

Treatment

There is no specific treatment for hepatitis B. Medications can be given to help relieve some of the symptoms. Other medications such as Interferon-α are available that may help slow the progression of the infection in a small number of patients.

Prevention

The best way to protect yourself is by getting vaccinated. Routine vaccination is now being done on everyone age eighteen and under. Vaccination is also recommended for those at high risk of getting hepatitis B.

High risk groups for hepatitis B include:[18]

- People who are having sex with infected persons
- IV drug users
- Homosexual men
- People with multiple sex partners or a sexually transmitted disease
- People who live with chronically infected persons
- Infants born to infected mothers
- Infants or children of immigrants from areas with high rates of hepatitis B infection (such as southeast Asia and sub-Saharan Africa)
- Health care and public safety workers
- Hemodialysis patients
- Patients who receive blood products

If you are not vaccinated and you do not have natural immunity from previous exposure, there are some things you can do to decrease your risk of infection:[19]

- If you are having sex, but not with one steady partner, use latex condoms correctly—every time you have sex. The efficacy of latex condoms in preventing infection with hepatitis B is unknown, but their proper use may reduce transmission.

- If you are pregnant, you should get a blood test for hepatitis B; infants born to infected mothers should be given hepatitis B immune globulin and vaccine within twelve hours after birth.
- Do not shoot drugs; if you shoot drugs, stop and get into a treatment program. If you don't stop, never share needles, syringes, water, or "works," and get vaccinated against hepatitis A and B.
- Do not share personal care items that might have blood on them (razors, toothbrushes).
- Consider the risks if you are thinking about getting a tattoo or body piercing. You might get infected if the tools have someone else's blood on them or if the artist or piercer does not follow good health practices and sterilize the equipment properly.
- If you currently have or have had hepatitis B, do not donate blood, organs, or tissue.
- If you are a health care or public safety worker, get vaccinated against hepatitis B, and always follow routine barrier precautions and safely handle needles and other sharp objects.

Most important, vaccination provides your best protection and you should consider it before becoming sexually intimate with any new partners. The vaccination is usually given as three separate injections over a six-month period. Adverse reactions are rare.

TRICHOMONIASIS

Trichomoniasis is a sexually transmitted infection caused by a protozoan parasite called *Trichomonas vaginalis*. An estimated five million people are infected with it each year in the United States.[20] It is spread by vaginal intercourse or by intimate contact from woman to woman.

Symptoms

Trichomonas most commonly infect the vagina of women and urethra in men. Many women with trichomoniasis have a yellow green vaginal discharge with a strong odor. There can be irritation and itching in the genital area that can cause some discomfort with intercourse. Men usually don't have symptoms and if they do, they have a mild discharge and some irritation or burning.

Most women have symptoms five to twenty-eight days after exposure. Having trichomoniasis may increase your risk of acquiring HIV if you are exposed to it. Trichomoniasis does not appear to cause any other long-term problems.

Diagnosis

Trichomoniasis is diagnosed by looking at the discharge under a microscope. The trichomonas organisms can be seen swimming in the discharge. Sometimes they can also be seen on a Pap smear.

Treatment

Antibiotics are used to treat trichomoniasis in both you and your partner(s).

Prevention

Your best protection against trichomoniasis is to use condoms every time you have intercourse.

HUMAN IMMUNODEFICIENCY VIRUS (HIV)

Human immunodeficiency virus or HIV is the sexually transmitted disease that people fear the most. Of all the sexually transmitted disease without a cure, HIV is the only one that has a high chance of killing you. Though medications are available to help slow the progression of the HIV infection, no cure is available. Approximately forty thousand Americans are infected with HIV a year.[21] Before you get too complacent and think it a disease that affects other people, homosexual men or young women, *an estimated 32 percent of women with AIDS were diagnosed with this disease when they were forty and over!*[22]

Though male-to-male sex and IV drug use have been the most common mode of spreading the disease, an increasing percentage of people are being infected by heterosexual contact. Vaginal, anal, or oral sex are all ways that HIV can be transmitted. The woman is more likely to become infected from sex (especially through vaginal and anal intercourse) with an infected man than vice versa. And sexual behaviors that increase the likelihood of trauma increase the risk of transmission of the virus. Oral sex with an infected male partner is probably a less frequent route of transmission of the virus, but is still possible.[23]

HIV can also be spread by transfusion of blood or blood products or from an infected mother to her baby during pregnancy, birth, or breast feeding. The HIV virus is spread through contact with blood, semen, vaginal fluid, breast milk, and other body fluids that contain blood. This occurs not only through physical intimacy, but also through occupational exposure, such as that faced by medical or public safety workers.

Once HIV gets into the body, it destroys certain white blood cells that are an important part of the immune system. Once the immune system is severely weakened, it is difficult for the body to fight off infections. If the infection cannot be controlled with medical intervention, this could lead to death.

Symptoms

Unfortunately, early in the infection, there are usually no symptoms. If someone has acquired the infection but has not been tested, they may unknowingly pass it on to others. Some people who know they have HIV will have unprotected sex with others because they don't care.

Diagnosis

HIV is detected by doing a blood test that checks for antibodies to HIV. The antibodies show up within six months of being infected with HIV. That means that your partner could test negative up to six months after exposure, though he may be infected. If you think you have been exposed, or wish be tested after being with a new partner, you should get tested immediately and again in six months, because it can take that long for the test to turn positive.

Treatment

There is no cure for HIV. Medications are available that slow its progression and help the body fight off infections. A very small number of people with HIV have not shown any signs of weakening of their immune systems, though the reason for this is unknown.

Prevention

The use of latex or polyurethane condoms can protect you against getting HIV, but is not completely safe. Semen is the main body fluid that can spread HIV during intercourse. Condoms keep the semen from coming in contact with your body, thus protecting you from the virus. However, condoms break, and there is the possibility of contact with other body fluids containing HIV. For example, if the man has an open sore in the genital area that is not covered by the condom, the virus could be transmitted by exposure to the bodily fluids coming from the sore.

Natural or lambskin condoms should not be used since HIV are small enough to pass through tiny openings in these condoms (those openings are too small for sperm to pass through, which is why they are still useful for birth control). Vaseline or oil-based lubricants should also be avoided because they can weaken the condom. Don't share sex toys, toothbrushes, razors, or needles.

SAFER SEX

The bottom line? There is no such thing as completely safe sex. Any sexual activity has risk. Using condoms during sex shouldn't be called "safe sex." This gives people the illusion that using condoms gives them a bulletproof shield against getting any disease. Instead, condom use should be called "*safer sex.*" Using condoms helps decrease the likelihood of certain sexually transmitted infections, but not all.

Women who have had a tubal ligation, hysterectomy, or have completely gone through menopause sometimes forget about condoms because they don't need birth control. But sexually transmitted infections can be found in men and women of all ages. Sex at any age can put you at risk for contracting these infections. Remember, almost a third of women were forty or older when they were diagnosed with AIDS. Condoms, though not perfect, are still your best friend and defense against these infections if you choose to become physically intimate with someone.

In the end, only you can decide if the risk of potential exposure to a sexually transmitted infection is worth the benefits of a sexual relationship.

DATE RAPE DRUGS

Women have always had to be cautious when meeting men or dating in the past because of the unknown. What is he like? Will we get along? Will we have things in common to talk about? What is he looking for—a quick fling or something more long term? What does he want from me? Should I go with a friend since I hardly know him? What should I do if he wants more physical intimacy than I'm ready for?

Now women have to be even more cautious because of the increasing availability and use of drugs such as GHB (gamma-hydroxybutyrate), Rohypnol (flunitrazepam), and others. Alcohol and other "recreational" drugs have been used to reduce a woman's inhibitions and defenses to make her more amenable to having sex. Often in these cases, women had a choice to use them or not, though men have raped women under the influence. With these new drugs, women don't even know they're ingesting them. Men use these hidden drugs specifically to rape.

GHB (gamma-hydroxybutyrate)

GHB is available as a powder or liquid and depresses the central nervous system. It can be easily produced from common ingredients using recipes available on the Internet. GHB is colorless and odorless, but may have a salty taste. At lower doses, it lowers inhibition and causes euphoria. At higher doses, it can cause drowsiness, dizziness, amnesia, confusion, hallucinations, nausea, vomiting, coma, and possibly death. These symptoms appear within fifteen minutes.[24]

Rohypnol (flunitrazepam)

Rohypnol is a powerful benzodiazepine (a drug in the same class as Valium and Xanax) that is odorless and tasteless when dissolved in a drink. It produces symptoms similar to alcohol intoxication within twenty to thirty minutes and may cause amnesia.[25]

These drugs are chosen because they are easily obtained, work quickly, reduce inhibitions, and cause amnesia while under its influence. Women who have been exposed to these drugs may feel unusually intoxicated after drinking only minimal amounts of alcohol. They may not remember anything that happens after the drug takes effect. Many times, victims wake up disoriented and may or may not recall if they have been sexually assaulted.

If You Think You're a Victim of Date Rape Drugs

If you suspect that you've been exposed to any of these drugs, you should save the first urine specimen you can get to be tested. Urine testing can detect these drugs, though GHB passes from the body very quickly and may not be detectable in your urine if you wait too long. You should also go to a rape treatment center to collect evidence of the sexual assault, to be tested and treated for possible sexually transmitted infections, and to prevent a possible pregnancy.

Tests for Date Rape Drugs

Coasters and cards are available that can test your drink for the presence of certain drugs such as GHB. However, they do not test for all the possible drugs used to facilitate sexual assault on women and can be falsely positive. One company does not recommend using its product with very acidic beverages such as drinks containing orange or grapefruit juices, milk products, crème or oily liquors, tonic water, or wines, which limits its usefulness.[26]

There are ways that you can stay safe when you go out:

- Go out with a friend. You can look out for each other and if something were to happen, you have someone who can safely take you home.
- Never leave your drink unattended. Take your drink with you if you have to go somewhere, even to the bathroom, and order a new one if yours has been left unattended.
- Don't accept drinks unless you watch it being made or poured.
- Drink slowly to avoid alcohol intoxication, and stop if you start to feel unusual in any way.
- If you get intoxicated very quickly or if you feel really sick, get help quickly. These drugs can be dangerous and possibly life threatening.
- If you use a coaster or card to test your drink, don't rely completely on the results since not all drugs are tested for and the test may give you a false negative or false positive result.

THE BOTTOM LINE

No matter how you look at it, being single again is fraught with many challenges. Though dating can be fun and meaningful, you need to be aware of the specter of sexually transmitted diseases. Also be wary of potential date rape drugs. As with everything else during these transitional periods, you need to be cautious and prudent.

CHAPTER 9

HORMONES
The Good, the Bad, and the Ugly

They're going to have to pry my hormones from my cold, dead hands.

—Kristy Miller

Hormones. Why have hormones become so embroiled in controversy?

A BRIEF HISTORY OF HORMONE THERAPY

*H*ormones have been used for decades to alleviate menopausal symptoms. Their use seemed intuitive: the decline of estrogen levels led to menopause. Giving women back estrogen would help their symptoms. A number of other problems also increased after menopause, including heart disease, osteoporosis, stroke, moodiness and irritability, memory problems, depression, Alzheimer's disease, cancers, and bladder and vaginal problems.

Could some of these problems be exacerbated by the loss of estrogen? And if so, could giving women estrogen after menopause help reduce the likelihood of these problems? It seemed possible, and if true, a major breakthrough in women's health would have been made. If only it were so simple. As with everything else in life, there is no free lunch and there is always more to something than meets the eye.

Is Menopause an Estrogen Deficiency Disease?

Some researchers began to look at menopause as a condition of estrogen deficiency, not unlike diabetes. In diabetes, your body does not make enough insulin, causing your blood sugar levels to rise to abnormal levels, leading to a number of problems. They felt that menopause was a disease of insufficient estrogen, which then caused the problems associated with menopause. They were motivated by a noble calling to help treat, through modern medicines, the discomfort and suffering caused by menopausal symptoms. Pharmaceutical companies also became interested in treating menopause, but from a business perspective. This led to the "medicalization" of menopause.

Some people began to look at menopause as a medical condition that could be treated with the use of hormones. And many women in the general public bought into this model because help was then only a pill away. We had pills to kill bacteria, as well as pills to help with pain, ulcers, depression, and anxiety, and even prevent pregnancy. And here was yet another pill to help ease women through menopause.

Not only did it lessen hot flashes and night sweats, but it also helped women sleep better, improved sexual functioning, improved women's skin, and held out the promise of preventing more serious problems such as heart disease, the number-one killer of menopausal women. It was almost like finding the fountain of youth—here was a pill that would make you look younger and keep you healthier.

This approach also led to the treatment of women who weren't having any problems with menopause. Some women go through menopause with minimal or no symptoms. Physicians reasoned that these women would also benefit from the long-term positive effects of the hormones such as the prevention of heart disease, osteoporosis, and vaginal atrophy. The logic is reasonable.

For example, high blood pressure is treated to prevent heart disease and strokes. Some people have symptoms when their blood pressure is high and so they are treated both for their symptoms and to prevent the future problems. But most people with high blood pressure have no symptoms and feel fine. But they need to be treated to prevent the future problems. Similarly, physicians thought that menopausal women would benefit from hormones.

Both Good and Bad Effects Have Been Discovered about Estrogen

As researchers delved more extensively into hormones and their effects on menopausal women, both benefits and risks were discovered. Estrogen did indeed help with hot flashes and night sweats. But estrogen used alone was found to increase the risk of endometrial cancer, a cancer of the lining of the uterus. So women who still had their uterus had to take a form of progesterone, the other female hormone, in order to prevent endometrial cancer. But other concerns regarding hormones became more worrisome, including estrogen's possible link to breast cancer, heart disease, strokes, blood clot formation in the deep veins of the legs, and gallbladder problems.

On the other hand, other beneficial aspects of estrogen were also being discovered, including: improvement in bone density and a decrease in osteoporosis, improvement of cholesterol levels, improvement of sexual functioning, fewer sleeping problems, and better skin elasticity (leading to fewer wrinkles). There were intimations that estrogen might prevent Alzheimer's disease, colon cancer, and tooth loss, and might also help with memory. Some of the information was conflicting. For example, some studies showed that estrogen decreased the risk of heart disease while others showed it increased it. So what are we supposed to believe?

The negative aspects of estrogen led to a backlash against the medical model of menopause. Many women and their physicians returned to the perspective that menopause is a natural stage of a woman's life (which it is) and does not need to be "treated" as if it were a disease (which it isn't). Other women began to look for alternatives to help them through this time of transition. Because of the negative press regarding estrogen or hormone replacement therapy, many women looked at hormones, especially estrogen, as bad, and were willing to try almost anything but estrogen to help with their symptoms.

Menopause and Puberty

So what is the right answer? Let's compare menopause to puberty. During puberty, there is a rise in hormone levels, leading to the changes of puberty. The physical changes are accompanied by mood swings, lapses in memory, and sleeping problems (adolescents want to stay up late and sleep late), yet we don't feel it necessary to "treat" these problems.

However, if there is a problem that is of sufficient concern, such as serious acne, severe mood swings, or clinical depression, then we inter-

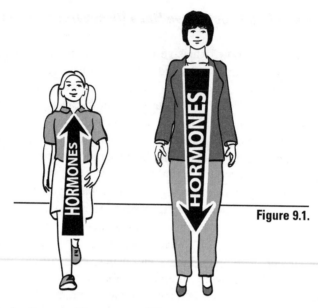

Figure 9.1.

vene. We don't treat all teenagers. We just treat the particular teenager for the problems that are having a significant impact on her life. Similarly, the menopausal transition is a very individual path. Many women will have minimal or no symptoms, thus needing no intervention. Others may have one issue or another that is causing significant distress for which they wish to find relief.

So perhaps a better way of looking at perimenopause and menopause is that it is a natural transition that women go through, like puberty, whose significant symptoms women may wish to treat. Estrogen is but one method to treat certain menopausal symptoms. Like any other therapy, it has its benefits and risks. It may not be the perfect solution but estrogen is still a reasonable option in the treatment of menopausal symptoms.

WHAT ARE HORMONES?

Hormones are chemicals made in one part of the body that affect cells in other areas of the body. Hormones act as messengers, carrying information and instructions that may have local or general effects. The female hormones are estrogen and progesterone, which are mainly produced by the ovaries. Androgens are considered the "male" hormones though women also produce small amounts of these hormones in the ovaries and adrenal glands (glands that are located on the top of the kidneys and produce hormones such as androgens, epinephrine, and cortisone).

ESTROGEN THERAPIES—
THE GOOD, THE BAD, AND THE UGLY

Estrogen, as noted, is primarily produced by the ovaries. Some estrogen is produced outside of the ovary by fatty tissue. Estrogen is responsible for developing the female reproductive system, for the changes seen during puberty, and for the stimulation of the lining of the uterus during the menstrual cycle. Estrogen also affects the bones, blood vessels, bladder, vagina, stomach, intestines, cholesterol levels, and skin.

Estrogen—The Good

Estrogen has been the main form of hormonal therapy to help with menopausal symptoms. There are different types of estrogen. The main forms of estrogen that women produce are estrone (E1), estradiol (E2), and estriol (E3). Each varies in its activity.

Estradiol is the most active estrogen in the body. Before menopause, estradiol is the main form of estrogen in a woman. It is the primary estrogen produced by the ovary. Estrone is a weak estrogen that is the most abundant estrogen after menopause. It is formed by other tissues in the body. Estriol is also a weak estrogen and is a breakdown product of estradiol and estrone.

There are currently no data to show that one of these forms of estrogen is better than the other when taken into the body by women. Until more studies are completed, all estrogens should be treated the same and assumed to have potentially similar risks and benefits. Most of the studies done to date have been done on conjugated equine estrogen (Premarin) and estradiol. Our understanding of risks and benefits of estrogen is based on this data.

Estrogen affects different parts of the body. Estrogen receptors have been found not only in the uterus, ovaries, vagina, and breast, but also in the brain, bone, skin, bladder, heart, gastrointestinal system, and liver. Estrogen receptors are structures on a cell to which estrogen attaches to affect that tissue. It is similar to a lock and key, where the estrogen receptor is the lock and estrogen is the key. When estrogen attaches to the receptor, it triggers a change in the cell. There are two known types of estrogen receptors. The number and types of these receptors found in different tis-

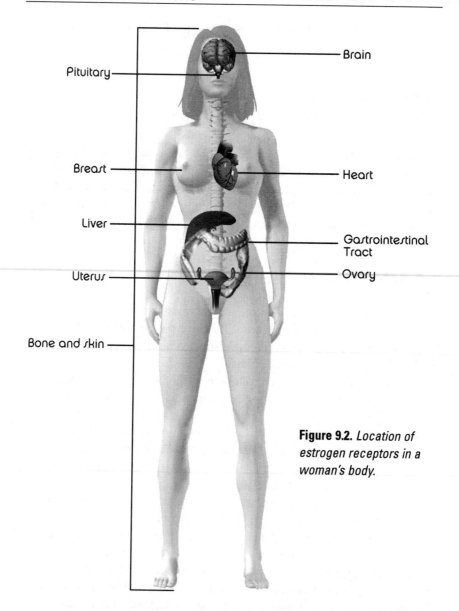

Pituitary

Brain

Breast

Heart

Liver

Gastrointestinal Tract

Uterus

Ovary

Bone and skin

Figure 9.2. *Location of estrogen receptors in a woman's body.*

sues may explain the positive and negative effects seen when estrogen or estrogen-like compounds are taken.

Estrogen has been shown to be helpful for a number of problems potentially faced by menopausal women including:

- Hot flashes
- Night sweats
- Insomnia
- Moodiness and irritability
- Vaginal dryness
- Painful intercourse
- Urinary tract infections
- Depressive symptoms
- Memory problems
- Tooth loss
- Osteoporosis
- Colon cancer

Estrogen may also be helpful for the following:

- Prevention of Alzheimer's disease
- Skin changes
- Urinary incontinence

Estrogen for Menopausal Symptoms

A large body of evidence supports the effectiveness of estrogen for treating hot flashes, night sweats, and atrophy of the genital area.[1] For these problems, estrogen is currently the most effective form of treatment. And it is for these problems that estrogen should be considered.

Estrogen helps significantly decrease the number and intensity of hot flashes and night sweats, which may be the way it helps with sleep problems and moodiness.[2] Estrogen also helps support the vagina through lubrication and elasticity. This, in turn, may help diminish sexual problems such as vaginal dryness and painful intercourse[3] and may also play a role in decreasing the risk of urinary tract infections.[4] Some studies suggest estrogen may also help with urinary incontinence.[5]

Estrogen and the Brain

Estrogen may have an effect on the brain. Besides helping with moodiness and irritability, estrogen may also help with memory,[6] decrease depressive symptoms,[7] and improve moods.[8] However, it is still unclear how much direct benefit estrogen may have on these areas and these benefits are still under debate. Estrogen may help with these problems by reducing night sweats thus improving sleep, which may ultimately uplift moods and improve memory.

There is also some evidence that estrogen may help reduce the risk of Alzheimer's disease or perhaps delay it.[9] However, once a woman has Alzheimer's disease, the use of estrogen does not seem to provide any benefit.[10] Estrogen may also help with balance, thus decreasing the possibility of falls and reducing the risk of fractures, which is very important as the bones get thinner with age.[11] These effects of estrogen on the brain are still unclear and should not be the primary reason to use estrogen at this time.

Estrogen and the Bones

Estrogen significantly improves bone density and decreases fractures. This may also be a major reason for less tooth loss with estrogen.[12] Teeth are attached to the jawbone and keeping this bone strong may help it hold onto teeth better. However, there are other options besides estrogen to help prevent and treat osteoporosis and bone loss. (See chapter 11 for more information on osteoporosis.) The risks and benefits of estrogen should be compared with the other options to determine which one makes the most sense.

Estrogen and Colon Cancer

Estrogen has been shown to decrease colon cancer, the third most common cancer in women.[13] Estrogen, though helpful, should not be used solely for this purpose since the other combined risks probably outweigh this benefit. Screening tests are available for colon cancer and should be used to detect it early. Dietary changes may also decrease the risk of colon cancer without the potential adverse effects of estrogen (see chapter 12).

Other Potential Benefits

Estrogen may help maintain skin thickness and elasticity and has been shown to decrease wrinkling and dryness.[14] Though this may sound mostly like a cosmetic benefit, this may also help with the healing of wounds. Still, this is a relatively minor benefit.

Estrogen—The Bad

Estrogen can have a number of side effects, including:

- Breast tenderness
- Vaginal bleeding
- Vaginal discharge
- Bloating
- Nausea
- Headache
- Fluid retention
- Moodiness
- Headache
- Hair loss
- Worsening of endometriosis

These side effects are in addition to its cost. Even with prescription drug coverage through insurance, purchasing these medications over many years can become expensive.

Like anything else, estrogen can have negative effects. Some women have no side effects with estrogen while others experience significant problems even on very low doses. Sometimes these side effects improve over time as the body gets used to the estrogen. Then again, the side effects may persist.

Unfortunately, there is no way to determine if you will have side effects ahead of time. Even if you had problems with birth control pills (which contain estrogen), you may not experience side effects because the amount of estrogen in pills used for menopause is generally much lower than that found in birth control pills.

Estrogen—The Ugly

And like many other things in life, there is a dark side to estrogen, the ugly side.

Estrogen now appears to increase the risk of:

- Blood clots in the deep veins in the leg (deep vein thrombosis)
- Heart attack
- Stroke

- Breast cancer
- High blood pressure (a rare idiosyncratic reaction)
- High triglycerides
- Gallbladder disease
- Endometrial cancer (only if taken without a progestin in women who still have their uterus)

The Women's Health Initiative (WHI) Study

The big story about hormones in 2002 was the premature discontinuation of one arm of the Women's Health Initiative (WHI) study. "Hormone Replacement Study a Shock to the Medical System" read one headline.[15] The study sent shock waves through the medical community as well as the millions of women taking hormones. What exactly was this study and what did it tell us?

The Women's Health Initiative (WHI) was a prospective, randomized, double-blinded study (the best kind of study; see chapter 10 for more information about different types of studies) of over sixteen thousand healthy women between the ages of fifty and seventy-nine who had gone through menopause. These women, who had not had a hysterectomy, were placed on estrogen and progestin—in the form of Prempro, a combination of conjugated equine estrogens (Premarin) and medroxyprogesterone acetate (Provera)—or placebo. Another arm of the study looked at over ten thousand postmenopausal women who had had a hysterectomy and placed them on estrogen alone—in the form of conjugated equine estrogens (Premarin)—or placebo.

The study was to follow these women for 8.5 years to determine the effect of these hormones on heart disease, stroke, deep vein thrombosis (blood clots in the deep veins in the legs), bone fractures, breast, uterine, and colon cancers. The study did not look at the effect of hormones on hot flashes or other menopausal symptoms.

One arm of the study looking at estrogen and progestin was halted about three years earlier than planned. This was mainly because researchers noted an increased risk of invasive breast cancer in the women who were taking estrogen and progestin. The study also showed that women taking these hormones had an increased risk of heart attack, stroke, and deep vein thrombosis. However, they had a decrease in colon cancer and fractures. But overall, the bad things outweighed the good in this group of women.

Though there was an increase in risk of adverse events, the overall risk was relatively low.

Health problem	Out of 10,000 women, the number of women taking placebo who would develop this problem in one year	Out of 10,000 women, the number of women taking the hormones who would develop this problem in one year	Difference per year out of 10,000 women
Breast cancer	30	38	8 more women with breast cancer
Heart attacks	30	37	7 more women with heart attacks
Strokes	21	29	8 more women with strokes
Blood clots	16	34	18 more women with blood clots
Colon cancer	16	10	6 fewer women with colon cancer
Hip fractures	15	10	5 fewer women with hip fractures

This study spread fear among menopausal women on hormones. Many women stopped taking them immediately. Others bombarded their physicians with worried phone calls. Some switched from Prempro, the medication in the study, to other hormone combinations.

What Did We Learn from This Study?

The WHI study reminded us that most things in life have a good and bad side. For many years, estrogen was thought to be the fountain of youth for women, helping them with menopausal symptoms and with numerous other positive health benefits. Though some of the negative effects were also known, this study helped clarify some of these risks.

The North American Menopause Society convened an advisory group in January 2003 and their recommendations included:[16]

- Treatment of menopause symptoms (hot flashes, vaginal dryness) remains the primary reason to use estrogen therapy

- Estrogen and progestin therapy should not be used to prevent heart disease.
- This data from the Women's Health Initiative cannot be directly applied to women in early menopause (before fifty years of age)
- Estrogen should be compared to the alternatives for the prevention of osteoporosis, by weighing the risks and benefits of each
- Use of hormones should be limited to the shortest duration while taking into consideration quality of life issues

The WHI study looked at one specific estrogen and progestin combination, Prempro. However, other combination hormone therapies, routes of administration (pill, patch, shot, etc.), or dosages should be considered to have the same risks until new data show any difference.

Lost in all this media attention is the other arm of the WHI looking at women who have had a hysterectomy and are taking estrogen only. This arm of the study is continuing because the risks and benefits are relatively balanced so far. Perhaps it is the addition of progestin that increases certain risks. This arm of the study is scheduled to end in 2005, at which time we will be able to determine what risks and benefits estrogen alone may have.

The American College of Obstetricians and Gynecologists recommends taking hormones for the shortest time and lowest dose that works for you. They also recommend that you have consultations with your physician at least once a year to review your reasons for taking hormones and to see if you can stop them.

So Is Estrogen Still an Option?

For women going through menopause, hormones are still an option for menopausal symptoms. It's not perfect and does have potential risks. But hormones are very effective at alleviating menopausal symptoms. Some women will not take them, nonetheless, because the risks are not worth the benefits. Many women will have only minimal symptoms and will not need even to consider hormones. But some women feel better on hormones and will wish to take them for their quality of life. However, they may still fear taking estrogen.

In reviewing the data from the WHI, women taking Prempro had a 26 percent higher chance of breast cancer. Sounds like a big increase, but that is the *relative risk* of getting breast cancer. In absolute numbers, eight more women out of ten thousand using Prempro would end up with breast cancer in a year. An increase, yes. And particularly from a public health standpoint where millions of women are taking this or a similar combination of hormones, the numbers are significant.

Also important to remember is that this applies only to women taking estrogen *and* progestins. The effects of estrogen alone are still being evaluated.

Those women who wish to take hormones and those who are having severe menopausal symptoms that nothing else has helped need to realize that although there is an increased risk, the chance that a given person on estrogen and progestin will have an adverse event is very low. Hormones are still a viable option.

Survey of Health Care Providers after the WHI Study

After the WHI study findings were released, a feeling of alarm spread through both the general public and the medical community. There were reports of women being told to stop their hormones by well-intentioned physicians. Expert panels of physicians and scientists convened to come to a consensus on the use of hormones. To determine what health care professionals were recommending in light of this new data, the authors did an informal survey to see what therapies are now being offered to perimenopausal and menopausal women.

Two hundred health care professionals (physicians, nurse practitioners, physician assistants, and certified nurse midwives) who treat perimenopausal and menopausal women from around the country completed the survey. Ninety-four percent would still offer hormone therapy for women with any symptoms related to menopause. The most common reasons they would prescribe hormones were for menopausal symptoms such as hot flashes (97 percent) followed by vaginal and bladder problems (72 percent), painful intercourse (62 percent), and prevention of osteoporosis (61 percent). Other common reasons for the use of hormones included the treatment of moodiness, insomnia, and treatment of osteoporosis related to menopause.

Slightly over 20 percent would still recommend hormones for women without menopausal symptoms for its potential benefits of preventing osteoporosis, colon cancer, and Alzheimer's disease.

Treatment options that these health care professionals would recommend other than hormones for women with symptoms going through menopause were exercise (97 percent), vitamins (74 percent), dietary changes (69 percent), antidepressants (67 percent), relaxation techniques (58 percent), and soy products (57 percent).

The results from this survey indicate that despite the concerns revealed by the WHI study, health care professionals are still prescribing hormones for menopausal women for a variety of reasons. These providers are now more carefully discussing the risks and benefits of hormone therapy with their patients. They are still offering it as an option for symptoms or medical problems caused by menopause when no other treatment has worked, tailoring therapy for the individual woman.

How Is Estrogen Given?

Estrogen can be taken as a pill, patch, ointments and creams applied to the skin, injection, pellet, vaginal creams, ring, or tablet. Currently, there is no evidence that one form of estrogen is superior to another.[17] Pills, patches, injections, and pellets are all ways of providing estrogen systemically, throughout the body. Estrogen given vaginally by creams, ring, or tablet not only acts locally on the vaginal tissues, but can also be readily absorbed through the vagina and go to the rest of the body.

Most studies have been done on estrogen pills. Currently, there is no evidence showing that giving estrogen in a form other than a pill is safer. However, an individual woman may do better on one preparation over another. For example, a woman may have difficulty absorbing the estrogen from her intestines for whatever reason and may do better with a patch.

The patch does not seem to increase triglycerides the way oral estrogen can, and may be an option for women with high triglyceride levels.[18] There is some intriguing data showing that the estrogen patch may provide some benefits not seen with the pill, but it is too early to tell if it will make a significant difference in improving overall health.[19]

For women with mostly vaginal symptoms, estrogen can be given locally, in the vagina. A very low-dose estrogen tablet can be used in the vagina and since the dose is so low, very little of the estrogen goes to the rest of the body. Even at this low a dose, improvement in vaginal symptoms can be seen.

Estrogen given as an injection or placed under the skin as a pellet can also be effective. The main concern is that estrogen levels can gradually rise as the estrogen builds up in the body, leading to significantly higher levels of estrogen than seen with pills. Given that the potential problems caused by estrogen may be related to how much is given, this is a cause for concern. Women who choose to use these forms of estrogen should have estrogen levels tested regularly.

Checking Estrogen Levels

Monitoring levels of estrogen is not as easy as it sounds. First, there are a number of ways estrogen levels can be measured in the blood, which can lead to differences in accuracy and reliability. The second problem is that there are different forms of estrogen. Not only are there the three main forms produced by the body—estradiol, estrone, and estriol—but there are also other forms of estrogen such as equine (horse) estrogens found in some of the estrogen formulations. Which ones should be checked?

Yet another problem is that most estrogen is bound to a protein called sex hormone binding globulin (SHBG) in the blood. The estrogen not bound to SHBG is called free estrogen, which is free to bind to estrogen receptors and affect the body. Anything that increases the SHBG decreases the amount of free estrogen. But when you check estrogen levels, you actually are determining the *total* estrogen level—this does not necessarily tell you how much *free* estrogen (the active form) is available, which is what you really want to know. For these reasons, checking estrogen levels is done occasionally in specific situations, but not on a routine basis.

Who Shouldn't Take Estrogen?

Women with the following conditions are at higher risk of adverse effects from estrogen and should carefully weigh the risks and benefits of estrogen before starting on them:

- History of breast cancer
- History of endometrial (uterine) cancer
- Unexplained vaginal bleeding
- Significant cardiovascular disease
- History of deep vein thrombosis or pulmonary embolus (a blood clot that goes to the lungs)
- Liver disease
- High triglycerides (detected by a lipid panel that checks different types of cholesterol and triglyceride levels)

Estrogen and Cancer

Estrogen can possibly stimulate breast and endometrial (uterine) cancers to grow. Women with a history of either of these cancers are generally advised not to take estrogen because of the concern that it may increase the risk of recurrence of these cancers. Women with unexplained vaginal bleeding may have endometrial cancer or endometrial hyperplasia, which are both stimulated by estrogen. The bleeding needs to be evaluated before estrogen is given (see chapter 3).

Estrogen and Cardiovascular Disease

Women with significant cardiovascular disease, such as a history of heart attack, stroke, bypass surgery, or angioplasty may be at higher risk of having more cardiovascular problems by taking estrogen. The WHI study showed an increased risk of heart attacks and strokes in women taking estrogen and progestin. Women should be warned of this risk before starting on hormones. Those with a history of cardiovascular disease should carefully weigh this increased risk against the benefit of estrogen and progestin before starting on hormone therapy. It is still unclear whether estrogen alone also has this effect.

Estrogen and Other Medical Problems

Women who have had a deep vein thrombosis (blood clot in the deep veins of the legs) or pulmonary embolus (blood clot that went to the lungs) are generally warned to avoid estrogen therapy. Estrogen increases these risks significantly.

Estrogen taken orally can increase triglycerides. Women with very high levels of triglycerides should be cautious about taking estrogen. Using the estrogen patch may avoid this negative effect, but that is not certain. Estrogen should also not be used in women with liver disease.

Which Form of Estrogen Is Best?

Estrogen is available in different forms. Conjugated equine estrogens, estradiol, ethinyl estradiol, estriol, estrone, esterified estrogens, estropipate, or synthetic conjugated estrogens—there are so many choices. If you choose to take estrogen, which one is better or safer than another? And with the recent concerns regarding hormones, many women are now looking for a "natural" estrogen to help with their symptoms. The question is, how do you define "natural"?

"Natural" Estrogens

Conjugated equine estrogen (more commonly known as Premarin) comes from pregnant mare's urine (thus it's name: **Pre**gnant **ma**re's **urin**e = Premarin). Now that's completely natural. Many of the other estrogen compounds available originally come from plants. Diosgenin is a plant steroid molecule that is extracted from yam or soy plants.[20] It is then chemically transformed in a laboratory into different estrogens, progestins, and androgens. But because the original substance comes from plants, it may be marketed as a "plant derived" or "natural" hormone.

So you could call most estrogens "natural," if you define it by where it originated, no matter how much it has been chemically altered. Premarin is not chemically altered since it is extracted from pregnant horse urine, so it is the closest to its natural origin.

Estradiol, Estrone, and Estriol

Others may say that Premarin is not "natural." Instead, natural is something chemically identical to what your body makes. Many women are now turning to compounding pharmacies (pharmacies that mix together special combinations of medications that are not commercially available) where estradiol, estrone, and estriol (those naturally found in the body) are mixed and put in a tablet to take. Triest is a combination of all three estrogens while biest has only estradiol and estriol. However, many women don't realize that estradiol, the most common estrogen found in the body, is commercially available alone at their local pharmacy with a prescription.

Since your body naturally makes these hormones, taking these should be safer—or so the reasoning goes. But the problem is that there is no study showing that any one of these estrogens is better than another or that taking them in ways that mimic the combination of estrogens in your body before menopause is safer than the way they are currently prescribed. Significant interest has been given to estriol as the "friendlier," more gentle estrogen. Estriol has been found to be effective in treating menopausal symptoms. Estriol is thought by some to have no effect on the lining of the uterus (thus not increasing the risk of uterine cancer) and not to increase the risk of breast cancer. However, no large long-term studies have been done on the safety of estriol.[21] Until more studies are done, estriol should be treated the same as the other estrogens.

So what to do? First, decide in consultation with your physician whether or not you really need hormones. If you want to take Premarin because it's the most studied estrogen available with the most data to show, that's one possibility. If you would rather take estradiol because it is biologically identical to what your body makes, that's another. If you want to take a compounded formulation because you feel it is more natural, that's yet another choice. And you may have to try different ones before you find one that fits you best. Some women do better on one form than another.

Don't be lulled into a false sense of security, however, that one form is significantly better or safer than another, because we currently don't have the data to support this. Perhaps in the future, we will find that one works better or is safer than another. Or we may find a synthetic form of estrogen that works only where we want it to, so that we can have the good without the bad. Only time will tell.

There are several hormone options available from the pharmacy listed in the table on the next page.

PROGESTERONE AND PROGESTINS

Progesterone is produced mainly by the ovaries with a small amount made by the adrenal gland. Progesterone helps support pregnancy and helps produce milk in breasts. Progesterone is also important in maintaining the menstrual cycle.

Why Do Women Have to Take Progesterone or Progestins?

Progestins (synthetic compounds that act like progesterone) and progesterone (which is chemically identical to that hormone made by your body) are mainly used to prevent endometrial cancer (cancer of the lining of the uterus) in women taking estrogen. As noted, estrogen given alone increases the risk of endometrial cancer.

Estrogen stimulates the endometrium, the lining of the uterus, to grow. Over time, the lining grows so much that it turns into endometrial hyperplasia (see chapter 3). If the lining continues to grow, it starts to grow out of control, becoming cancerous.

Compare it to a lawn. Estrogen is like a nutrient stimulating the grass to grow. If you keep adding nutrients, the grass grows and grows and becomes very high, which is what happens when you have hyperplasia. Hyperplasia basically means that something is overgrowing. If this con-

Available Estrogen, Progestin, and Androgen Products

Estrogen pills

Cenestin	synthetic conjugated estrogens
Estrace	estradiol
Estratab	esterified estrogens
Gynodiol	estradiol
Menest	esterified estrogens
Ogen	estropipate (piperazine estrone sulfate)
Ortho-Est	estropipate (piperazine estrone sulfate)
Premarin	conjugated equine estrogens

Progestin pills

Amen	medroxyprogesterone acetate
Aygestin	norethindrone acetate
Cycrin	medroxyprogesterone acetate
Megace	megestrol acetate (not for uterine protection)
Micronor	norethindrone
Nor-QD	norethindrone
Ovrette	norgestrel
Prometrium	progesterone USP (in peanut oil)
Provera	medroxyprogesterone acetate

Estrogen plus progestin pills

Activella	estradiol and norethindrone acetate
Femhrt	ethinyl-estradiol and norethindrone acetate
Ortho-Prefest	estradiol and norgestimate
Premphase	conjugated equine estrogens and medroxyprogesterone acetate
Prempro	conjugated equine estrogens and medroxyprogesterone acetate

Estrogen plus testosterone pills

Estratest and Estratest HS	esterified estrogens and methyltestosterone

Estrogen patches

Alora	estradiol
Climara	estradiol
Esclim	estradiol
Estraderm	estradiol
FemPatch	estradiol
Vivelle; Vivelle-Dot	estradiol

Estrogen plus progestin patch

CombiPatch	estradiol and norethindrone acetate

Estrogen vaginal

Estrace Cream	micronized 17-beta-estradiol
Estring	estradiol
Femring	estradiol acetate
Premarin Cream	conjugated equine estrogens
Vagifem	estradiol

tinues, then you have the beginnings of cancer: cells growing out of control and spreading to other parts of the body.

So women who have their uterus need to take progesterone. Progesterone and progestins are given orally, vaginally, or as an intrauterine device. Progesterone keeps the uterine lining from growing or can be used to make the uterine lining slough off. Progesterone is necessary to prevent the formation of endometrial hyperplasia and cancer in women taking estrogen.

How Is Progesterone Taken?

Taking progesterone ten to fourteen days a month essentially mimics the time before a period. When the progesterone is stopped, there is a drop in progesterone levels. This triggers the uterine lining to be released, which you see as your period. The bleeding usually starts two to three days after you stop taking the progesterone. Bleeding will be seen only if there is enough estrogen (either made by the body or taken as a medication) to stimulate the lining of the uterus to grow. The progesterone protects you from hyperplasia or cancer by regularly cleaning out the uterine lining.

Progesterone can also be taken continuously. In this case, a smaller amount of progesterone is taken every day. The progesterone suppresses the growth of the uterine lining, which counters the effect of the estrogen. When estrogen and progesterone are taken daily, most women eventually have no further bleeding. No bleeding is the practical advantage of taking daily estrogen and progesterone, making this option for hormone treatment much more attractive. How many women want periods if they don't have to have them? Still, some women continue to have bleeding on this regimen. The problem is not just one of inconvenience, but of trying to determine the cause of the bleeding.

Most vaginal bleeding after menopause is benign. But the main sign of endometrial (or uterine) cancer is uterine bleeding. About 9 percent of women in their fifties with postmenopausal bleeding will have endometrial cancer and the risk increases with advancing age.[22] (See chapter 3 for more information on endometrial hyperplasia and cancer.)

What Other Effects Does Progesterone Have on the Body?

Progesterone affects other parts of the body besides the uterus. In fact, progesterone and progestins may act differently in different parts of the body. There is no data showing that they protect against breast cancer and now there is some concern that they may possibly promote it. They may help with bone strength and menopausal symptoms, though not as effectively as estrogen.[23]

The side effects of progestins and progesterone include:

- Breast tenderness
- Fluid retention
- Rash
- Acne
- Unwanted hair growth
- Hair loss
- Headache
- Mood swings and irritability
- Sleepiness
- Possibly promotes breast cancer

Most of these side effects, with the exception of breast cancer promotion, are generally mild, although they may be severe in some women.

What about Progesterone Cream?

The effects of progesterone and progestins, which are given orally or vaginally, are described above. Progesterone cream has been touted as a safer alternative to estrogen because it is natural. However, it is the same as the progesterone that was described earlier, but taken by a different route. The cream is applied to the skin where it is absorbed by the body. Progesterone cream has been promoted as a way to help improve mood, reduce menopausal and premenstrual symptoms, and improve bone strength with very few side effects.

Unfortunately, the majority of the studies don't support these claims. This is probably because very little of the progesterone is actually absorbed. Studies looking at women using various doses of progesterone cream showed only a slight increase in blood levels of progesterone. When compared to placebo, progesterone cream did not improve menopausal symptoms, moods, or sexual feelings.[24] There are also no studies supporting the use of progesterone cream to help strengthen bone or to protect against endometrial cancer in women taking estrogen.

Despite the hype, the benefits seen with progesterone cream may be due to the placebo effect. Some women using progesterone cream believe it to be helpful, however. Until more information is available, there does not seem to be any significant benefit to using progesterone cream.

TESTOSTERONE

Do Testosterone and Other "Male" Hormones Have a Role in Women?

As stated earlier, androgens are "male" hormones, but women also make these hormones in much smaller amounts. They are produced by the ovaries and adrenal glands. Androgens include testosterone and androstenedione. They contribute to your sex drive, build up your bones and muscles, and enhance your feeling of general well-being (for more information on testosterone and libido, see chapter 6).

Testosterone Levels Change with Age

A large part of the testosterone in a woman is produced by the ovaries. As you grow older, your testosterone levels gradually decrease. Testosterone levels in women at forty are about half those of women in their early twenties.[25] However, testosterone levels don't drop as quickly as estrogen when you go through menopause. Testosterone levels gradually decrease over time even during and after menopause.

Taking Testosterone: Its Effect in Women

In women who have had their ovaries removed, testosterone has been shown to be helpful with libido and moods. However, in women going through menopause who still have their ovaries, the role of testosterone supplementation is less clear. There is some evidence showing testosterone supplementation may improve some aspects of sexual function, muscle mass and strength, mental function, and sense of well-being, though the studies are inconsistent.[26]

Adding testosterone to estrogen seems to improve bone density more than when estrogen is used alone and also helps menopausal symptoms that are not responsive to estrogen alone.[27] However, the amount needed to achieve these benefits and the long-term safety and consequences of using testosterone in women are still unknown.

Despite these uncertainties, some women may want to try testosterone for a variety of reasons. If you and your physician choose testosterone for you, you should have blood levels checked to make sure the testosterone level doesn't get too high. Remember, there are potential side effects of testosterone including increased hair growth, hair loss, acne, oily skin, deepening of the voice, bloating, fluid retention, and liver problems. Testosterone may also have a negative effect on cholesterol levels and the heart.[28] As noted, these side effects are generally reversible once the testosterone is discontinued except for the deepening of the voice (which may be important if you are a singer).

Over-the-Counter Androgens: DHEA and Androstenedione

DHEA (dihydroepiandrosterone) and androstenedione are available without prescription over the counter. They have been classified as dietary supplements and are therefore not tightly regulated like other medications. DHEA has been hyped in the media to help with a myriad of health problems such as improving the immune system, improving mood and energy, and boosting sex drive.

Both of these androgens can increase testosterone and estrogen levels in women.[29] So these androgens could possibly help you feel better, but they are probably doing it by increasing hormone levels in your body. And that is why you have to be just as cautious with these over-the-counter choices as you do with any other hormone you may choose to take. In fact, you need to be more cautious because of the lack of quality control (see chapter 10). These supplements have not been subjected to long-term testing and may have other negative side effects.

SERM (SELECTIVE ESTROGEN-RECEPTOR MODULATOR)

What Is a SERM (Selective Estrogen-Receptor Modulator)?

SERMs (*selective estrogen-receptor modulators*) act like estrogens in certain areas of the body and like antiestrogens in others. The two main SERMs available in this country are tamoxifen (Nolvadex) and raloxifene (Evista).

Tamoxifen is well known for treating breast cancer. It can also reduce the risk of breast cancer in women who are at higher risk for it. However, tamoxifen worsens hot flashes and increases the risk of uterine cancer and deep venous thrombosis (blood clots in the deep veins of the legs that cause pain and swelling in the leg).

Raloxifene improves bone density, protecting against osteoporosis; it also decreases LDL, the bad cholesterol, but not quite as well as estrogen. There is some evidence that raloxifene may even help protect the heart but a more definitive answer will be made when the results of the Raloxifene Use in the Heart (RUTH) trial is completed. Raloxifene also decreases the risk of breast cancer and does not increase the risk of uterine cancer.

Raloxifene is approved for the prevention and treatment of post-menopausal osteoporosis. It is not as effective as estrogen or the bisphos-phonates (Fosamax and Actonel). (For more information about the treatment of osteoporosis and bisphosphonates, see chapter 11.) Because clinical trials have shown that raloxifene decreases fractures of the spine but not of the hip, it is probably most beneficial for women with primarily osteoporosis of the spine.

Raloxifene does have the added benefit of decreasing breast cancer. The STAR (Study of Tamoxifen and Raloxifene) trial will determine how effectively raloxifene prevents breast cancer in high-risk women and if it should be used for this. Raloxifene is a reasonable option for post-menopausal women who wish to protect their bones and who don't have significant hot flashes.[30]

Raloxifene does have some side effects, including:

- Increased hot flashes
- Leg cramps
- Fluid retention and swelling
- Deep venous thrombosis (blood clots in the legs)
- Pulmonary embolus (blood clots that go to the lungs and can be life threatening)

Women who are at increased risk of forming blood clots in their veins should avoid raloxifene. Surgery or prolonged immobilization such as sitting on long flights may increase the risk of deep venous thrombosis. Because raloxifene also increases this risk, ideally, it should be discontinued before surgery or long flights.

Some of the studies with SERMs have followed subjects for over five

Comparison of Actions and Side Effects of Estrogen and SERMs[31]

Side Effect	Estrogen	Raloxifene	Tamoxifen
Hot flashes	↓↓↓	↑	↑
Uterine bleeding	↑↑↑	↔	↑
Risk of endometrial cancer	↑↑*	↔	↑
Prevention of postmenopausal bone loss	↑↑↑	↑↑	↑
Risk of breast cancer	↑↑	↓↓	↓↓
Favorable pattern of serum lipids	↑↑↑	↑	↑
Venous thrombosis	↑↑	↑↑	↑↑

↔ no change	↑ increased effect	↓ decreased effect

* This effect can be prevented by using progestins with estrogen

years and no other adverse effects have been found to date. There are currently several large-scale, long-term studies being done on SERMs to determine other risks and benefits of this class of medications. To determine the length of time to stay on these medications, you will need to discuss it with your physician.

THE BOTTOM LINE

They used to call giving hormones to postmenopausal women "hormone replacement therapy," as if there was something missing and had to be given back. Hormones don't need to be replaced in a woman going through menopause. The drop in hormone levels is the normal, natural state of affairs at this time of life.

Hormones can still provide benefit to a woman during perimenopause and menopause. However, hormones, whether they are prescribed by your physician or bought as a supplement from a natural food store, should be viewed in the same light as any other medical intervention. You should have a clear idea of why you are taking them, what benefits they provide, and whether the potential risks are worth those benefits. Estrogens are no longer viewed as the fountain of youth, but neither should they be vilified and relegated to eternal damnation.

CHAPTER 10

NATURAL REMEDIES
What They Don't Tell You

*M*any women have been interested in turning to "natural" or alternative remedies to help them with various menopausal problems, believing them to be effective and safer than medications. With new studies showing risks for different medications, especially hormones, coming out so frequently, many women are considering what they feel is a safer alternative to ease their symptoms. "Hormones scare me." "It's natural so it must be safer." "Menopause is a natural process so I want to use natural remedies." "St. John's Wort for depressive symptoms." "Black cohosh for hot flashes." "Vitamin E for breast pain." What are "natural" remedies? How do they work? Are they safe? Do they help?

WHAT IS COMPLEMENTARY AND ALTERNATIVE MEDICINE?

First of all, how do we define complementary and alternative medicine? The best way is to first define conventional medicine. Conventional medicine is commonly considered to be medicine that is generally taught, practiced, and accepted by medical doctors, doctors of osteopathy, respected medical schools, and other health professionals such as registered nurses, psychologists, and physical therapists. Complementary and alternative medicine would then be treatments, therapies, and practices that are currently not part of the conventional Western medical system.

Complementary and alternative therapies have not been adopted by conventional medicine mainly due to a lack of well-designed scientific studies showing their effectiveness and safety in treating various medical conditions. Some people may argue that rigid scientific studies are not necessary because some of these therapies have had a long history of safe and effective use. But how safe are they? Often we really don't know. Many times, short- and long-term problems may not be discovered unless formal testing is done.

If an alternative treatment seems to be helpful, then it can be studied further to see if it is truly helpful and to determine what side effects it may have. Many conventional treatments were discovered this way. But without further study, it would be difficult to determine exactly how much a given treatment may help, what the proper amount to give should be, and what its short- and long-term safety is.

Complementary medicine is used together with, or in complement to, conventional medicine. For example, some people may use hypnotherapy along with pain medicines to help them control pain. Alternative medicine is used in place of conventional medicine. An example would be the use of herbs to treat severe diabetes (something we would not recommend) instead of insulin and diet as recommended by a physician.

However, just because it is currently not part of our current medical system does not necessarily mean that it is ineffective or useless. Complementary and alternative forms of medicine may become part of conventional medicine once reliable studies become available as to the efficacy and safety of a particular alternative treatment.

The National Center for Complementary and Alternative Medicine (part of the National Institutes of Health) classifies complementary and alternative therapies into five categories.[1]

1. **Alternative Medical Systems.** Alternative medical systems are built upon complete and complex systems of theory and practice. Often, these systems have evolved apart from and earlier than the conventional medical approach used in the United States. Examples of alternative medical systems that have developed in Western cultures include homeopathic medicine and naturopathic medicine. Examples of systems that have developed in non-Western cultures include traditional Chinese medicine and Ayurveda.

2. **Mind-Body Interventions.** Mind-body medicine uses a variety of techniques designed to enhance the mind's capacity to affect bodily function and symptoms. Some techniques that were considered complementary and alternative medicine in the past have become mainstream (for example, patient support groups and cognitive-behavioral therapy). Other mind-body techniques are still considered complementary and alternative medicine, including meditation, prayer, mental healing, and therapies that use creative outlets such as art, music, or dance.

3. **Biologically Based Therapies.** Biologically based therapies in complementary and alternative medicine use substances found in nature, such as herbs, foods, and vitamins. Some examples include dietary supplements, herbal products, and the use of other so-called natural but as yet scientifically unproven therapies (for example, using shark cartilage to treat cancer).

4. **Manipulative and Body-Based Methods.** Manipulative and body-based methods in complementary and alternative medicine are based on manipulation and/or movement of one or more parts of the body. Some examples include chiropractic or osteopathic manipulation, and massage.

5. **Energy Therapies.** Energy therapies involve the use of "energy fields." They are of two types:

- *Biofield therapies* are intended to affect energy fields that they presume surround and penetrate the human body. The existence of such fields has never been scientifically proven. Some forms of energy therapy supposedly manipulate biofields by applying pressure and/or manipulating the body by placing the hands in, or through, these fields. Examples include gi gong, Reiki, and Therapeutic Touch.
- *Bioelectromagnetic-based therapies* involve the unconventional use of electromagnetic fields, such as pulsed fields, magnetic fields, or alternating current or direct current fields.

Use of Complementary and Alternative Medicines among Perimenopausal Women

A wide variety of complementary and alternative therapies are available. According to the North American Menopause Society, more than 30 percent of women use herbal supplements, "natural" estrogen, plant estrogens, or acupuncture. In 1997, an estimated $27 billion was spent for alternative therapies in this country.[2] Why do so many people turn to alternative medicine for help? For some, it is a distrust or dissatisfaction with conventional medicine. For others, alternative medicines fit more closely with their personal belief system.

The question thus becomes, What is effective and safe for a woman going through perimenopause?

For the treatment of hot flashes a number of complementary and alternative therapies have been promoted as being helpful, including:

- Black Cohosh (*Cimicifuga racemosa*)
- Dietary Soy
- Phytoestrogens
- Dong Quai (*Angelica sinensis*)
- Chaste Tree Berry (*Vitex agnus-castus*)
- Flaxseed
- Evening Primrose Oil (*Oenothera biennis*)
- Red clover
- Ginseng (*Panax ginseng*)
- Acupuncture
- Deep Breathing
- Vitamin E

We will explore how effective these remedies really are.

EVALUATING ALTERNATIVE MEDICINES

How effective are these alternative remedies? By evaluating studies that have been published, we can get an idea as to the efficacy of different treatment options. However, not all studies are equal. Some studies are poorly done and may give misleading results.

A number of problems can affect the outcome of a study, including:

- Researcher bias
- Patient bias
- Number of subjects

- Differences between the treated and untreated groups
- Prospective versus retrospective study
- Placebo response

Researcher Bias in a Study

Researcher bias can be a problem because if the researcher knows who gets what treatment, he or she may unknowingly skew the results by the way questions are asked or how the patient is evaluated. For example, if the researcher gives the patient a treatment he or she believes to be effective, the follow-up question may be asked in a way that leads the patient to give answers the researcher wants to hear. Instead of asking, "Was the treatment effective and if so, how effective was it?" the question may be posed as, "How effective was your treatment?" implying that the treatment is effective. The answers will then tend to be more positive.

Patient Bias in a Study

Patient bias may affect a study because if a patient knows what she is getting, it may affect how she feels. For example, a patient may be treated and believe that the treatment is either effective or ineffective. Her belief that the treatment will or won't work may affect her assessment of the treatment and skew the results. That's why a blinded study, where the patient is unaware if they are in the active treatment group or the placebo group, is important. A placebo is basically something given in a study that looks like the active product but contains only an inert substance such as sugar.

A double-blinded study is one where both the researcher and the patient are unaware of which treatment group the patient is in. This type of study helps reduce researcher and patient bias as factors that may affect the outcome of a study.

Number of Subjects

In studies with a small number of subjects, having an improvement in only a few subjects can make it seem like a treatment has a bigger impact than it really does. To give an extreme example, if there was a study with only one subject and the person treated improves, it looks like there is a 100 percent response to the treatment. The larger the study, the more likely the result will not be due to chance.

Differences between the Treated and Untreated Groups

Differences between the treated and untreated groups may make the treatment appear effective when in fact it is the difference between the groups rather than the intervention that explains the findings in a study. For example, if a treatment were to address muscle strength and the treated group was fitness trainers while the untreated group was in poor health, then it may appear that the treatment was effective. However, it was the difference in the groups, not the treatment, that probably explained the improvement.

Prospective versus Retrospective Studies

A prospective study is one in which a study is started and the subjects are followed over time. At the beginning of a prospective study, the researchers determine what treatment they will try and what outcomes they will follow over the course of the study. They can then see if their treatment helps. For example, if you wanted to study the effect of a medication on hot flashes, you would have half the subjects take the medicine and half not, to see if it helps.

In retrospective studies, you start with the subjects who have a problem and look backward in time to see if there is a difference between the subjects with the problem and those without it. If there is a difference, that may be a reason for the problem. But you can't be sure if there isn't another reason that you didn't find in the study to explain the difference. Prospective studies are generally considered more reliable whereas retrospective studies usually give you a good place to start to determine the cause of a problem.

The Placebo Response

The best way to find out if a treatment is effective is to look at studies that have compared a remedy to placebo. As noted above, a placebo is basically something given in a study that looks like the active product, but contains only an inert substance such as sugar. Comparing a remedy to placebo is important. Many times, when a person is given a pill and told that it will help with her problem, she will actually feel better. This is called the placebo effect.

The placebo effect occurs because a person's belief in something actually helps them get better. And if someone is handed a pill in a clinical environment or takes one based on seeing an ad, he or she will often believe it is helpful. A person's response to placebo usually diminishes over time, however. Also, just because someone responds to a placebo does not mean that the problems are only in that person's head. It just shows that the mind can have a powerful effect over symptoms.

Most studies show a placebo response in 20 to 30 percent of women with menopausal symptoms when given a placebo.[3] So any study that shows that a particular therapy works for symptoms such as hot flashes always needs to be compared with placebo. This way, we can know if the therapy is more effective than placebo. If it is not, then it is the power of suggestion that is helping with the symptom, not the actual therapy itself. And if you are going to spend money on a remedy (and these alternative remedies can be quite expensive), you would like to know that it is more effective than sugar pills. You also want to know that it can't hurt you.

This is why you have to be careful with what is called anecdotal experience. A friend or even a health care professional may tell you that something helped them or a patient. They may actually feel better, but it could be the placebo effect at work. We will look at different alternative treatment options and the studies that have compared them to placebo.

BOTANICAL OR HERBAL REMEDIES

Remedies derived from plants have become one of the most popular alternatives women have turned to for treatment of their menopausal symptoms. These remedies are touted as being safer because they are "natural." Recall that many poisons, such as certain mushrooms, plants, and berries, are "natural." "Natural" does not necessarily mean safe or helpful.

We will review the information available regarding many of these remedies. Keep in mind that over half of the medications prescribed originally come from natural sources. Aspirin is from the bark of willow trees (*Salix alba*). Codeine and morphine comes from poppy seeds (*Papaver somniferum*). Digoxin is a heart medicine from foxglove (*Digitalis purpurea*). Taxol, used for chemotherapy, comes from the Pacific Yew tree (*Taxus brevifolia*).

Are herbal and botanical remedies safe? Maybe yes, but maybe not. Think of it this way. If you took willow bark and concentrated it and made it into a pill, it may help your pain, similar to aspirin. After all, that's where aspirin originated. But if you took an extract from the Pacific Yew tree, you could potentially be taking the active ingredient in Taxol, a drug used for cancer chemotherapy. So herbal or botanical remedies may very well be effective, but they may also be very powerful and potentially very dangerous.

Many people are under the impression that these herbal and botanical remedies are thoroughly tested for safety and effectiveness. Unfortunately, this is not the case. These remedies are now regulated by the Dietary Supplement Health and Education Act of 1994 (DSHEA), which does not adhere to the rigorous standards held for medicines.

What Is a Dietary Supplement?

The Dietary Supplement Health and Education Act of 1994 defined dietary supplements as: (1) a vitamin, (2) a mineral, (3) an herb or other botanical, (4) an amino acid, (5) a dietary supplement used to supplement the diet by increasing the total dietary intake, or (6) a concentrate, metabolite, constituent, extract, or combination of any of the above ingredients.

Aren't Dietary Supplements Proven to Help as Advertised?

Most people believe that dietary supplements such as herbs, vitamins, and minerals are closely regulated to ensure that they are safe and effective for treating problems as advertised. Unfortunately, this is not necessarily true.

The companies manufacturing these dietary supplements are now responsible for determining their safety and effectiveness. Nevertheless, they do *not* have to provide the FDA with evidence to substantiate this before or after they market their products. A dietary supplement cannot claim to cure, treat, or prevent disease without prior FDA approval. However, the manufacturer can make vague nondisease claims such as "for hot flashes," "promotes relaxation," "helps maintain a healthy circulatory system," and "supports the immune system," which to most people sound like medical benefits.[4]

Much of the use of dietary supplements is based on past experience— *not* on rigorous scientific study. So far, many of the studies have been poorly done with no placebo control group to rule out the placebo effect (see above). More recent studies are better done, but there are still hurdles to overcome, such as consistency of the supplement used. Even if one brand is shown to be helpful, that cannot be generalized to different brands of that supplement because of differences in how they are grown, what parts of the plant are used, and how they are processed, to name a few. Even within one company, there is no assurance that one batch of supplement is of the same quality as another.

How Are Dietary Supplements Monitored?

Unlike pharmaceutical companies, manufacturers and distributors of dietary supplements are not required by law to record, investigate, or forward to the FDA any reports they receive of injuries or illnesses that may be related to the use of their products. If a dietary supplement is found to be unsafe, it is up to the FDA to prove this before they can restrict or remove the product from the market. A medicine, in contrast, cannot be sold until it has passed a long and stringent series of tests.[5]

One example is kava, an herbal supplement sold as a "tension relaxer" that has been linked to liver damage and failure. Because of the evidence, its sale has been banned in Canada, Singapore, the United Kingdom, and other European nations. The Medicines Control Agency in the United Kingdom stated, "There is clear evidence linking kava-kava with rare cases of liver toxicity."[6] They further stated, "Investigators have been unable to identify factors that would predict which individuals are at risk of adverse reactions." Their conclusion: "There is no evidence to support a safe dose of kava." However, kava is still available in the United States because the FDA must first collect enough data to prove kava is unsafe before it can ban the sale of this dietary supplement.

But Aren't Dietary Supplements Manufactured According to Strict Guidelines?

There are currently no FDA regulations specific to manufacturing dietary supplements that establish minimum standards. This has led to a wide variation in the quality of dietary supplements available in this country. The two main problems with this lack of standardization are: (1) a discrepancy between the amount of the active ingredients as listed on the label and the actual amount in the product itself and (2) adulteration or contamination of the product.

Analyses of "standardized" herbal preparations show that botanical products often do not contain the amount of the compound stated on the label. An analysis of twenty ephedra supplements from different companies showed that the actual content of the different active ingredients compared to what was stated on the label varied widely. Some had very little of the stated ingredients while others had over 150 percent of the label claim. One product had over 100 percent difference in the amount of one active ingredient from one lot to the next.[7]

The second problem is adulteration or contamination of the dietary supplement. Over five hundred Chinese patent medicines were screened for the presence of heavy metals such as lead, mercury, arsenic, and 134 other drugs. About 10 percent were found to contain undeclared drugs or toxic levels of metals.[8] Some of these contaminants may be a byproduct of the manufacturing process, while others such as drugs might have been added in the hopes of improving the effectiveness of the dietary supplement.

Plants and Herbs Are Complex

St. John's wort, which some people take for depression, contains naphtho-dianthrones (hypericin and pseudohypericin), phloroglucinols (hyperforin and adhyperforin), phenylpropanes, flavonol derivatives, biflavones, proan-thocyanidins, xanthones, and amino acids. Which ingredient or combination of ingredients is responsible for its action is still unclear. Plants and herbs are very complex with a multitude of potentially beneficial or harmful components. Processing a plant or herb to be used as a dietary supplement exposes the consumer to a number of different substances.

This also makes these supplements difficult to study. For example, originally, it was thought that the hypericin in St. John's wort was the active ingredient that helped with depression. So this was what is measured and placed on the labels of this product guiding the amount to take. However, more recently, the focus has shifted to hyperforin as the major active component. This means that the use of hypericin to guide therapy may have been incorrect. Even if two brands of St. John's wort have the same amount of hypericin, they may differ in the amount of hyperforin.

Trying to figure out which component is the active one makes it more complicated to study. Each brand may have varying amounts of the different components depending on where their plants are grown and how they are processed.

But They're Natural, So They're Safe

As noted earlier, many "natural" substances are poisonous. You don't have to look farther than your backyard to find things like poison mushrooms that can be lethal if eaten. Another concern is that these natural plants and herbs are being highly concentrated and ingested in a way that is different from their past use.

Take the coca leaf, for example. For thousands of years it had been used by natives in South America as a mild stimulant similar to coffee when the leaves were chewed. However, when the coca leaves were taken and concentrated, one of the constituents isolated was cocaine. In this highly concentrated form, cocaine causes a number of effects that were not seen when taken in its original form in the leaf.

If you think about it, many of the medicines we use now were discovered in a similar fashion. A plant that was found to have certain properties was studied and the different components were isolated and tested to see which one caused the desired effect. It was then tested and studied to determine the proper dose and side effects. It's not a perfect system because harmful medications are sometimes approved, but it does help minimize the likelihood of danger.

Supplements may also interact with other medications. The components of supplements may increase or decrease the effectiveness of other medications. For example, St. John's wort has been shown to cause blood levels of certain medications to fall to subtherapeutic levels, leading to potentially serious adverse effects.[9] Often people forget to tell their physician that they are taking herbal supplements when asked what medications they are on. It is important to let your physician know all the medications *and* supplements you take even though serious interactions between supplements and medications are not always known.

The Bottom Line on Dietary Supplements

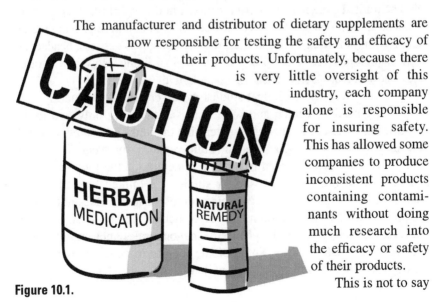

The manufacturer and distributor of dietary supplements are now responsible for testing the safety and efficacy of their products. Unfortunately, because there is very little oversight of this industry, each company alone is responsible for insuring safety. This has allowed some companies to produce inconsistent products containing contaminants without doing much research into the efficacy or safety of their products.

This is not to say

Figure 10.1.

that all dietary supplements are unsafe or harmful. Potentially, some may be beneficial, but you can't be sure. Others are possibly ineffective, leading you to spend money for no benefit. And any number are most likely harmful. As for dietary supplements, the problems at this time are to figure out what supplement is actually helpful and which companies are producing a quality product. Caveat emptor. "Let the buyer beware" has never been so true.

BOTANICAL OR HERBAL REMEDIES FOR MENOPAUSAL SYMPTOMS

Black Cohosh (Cimicifuga racemosa)

Black cohosh is an herb from the root of a plant used by Native Americans and Europeans for a number of gynecological problems including hot flashes, menstrual cramping, and PMS. It is one of the top-selling menopausal herbal remedies in Germany.

How black cohosh works is unknown. The German Commission E Monographs indicate that black cohosh acts like an estrogen, binding to estrogen receptors.[10] Some researchers do not agree with this and feel that black cohosh works, if indeed it does, through some other mechanism.

The limited evidence that exists is mixed in the use of black cohosh for menopausal symptoms. One study showed some benefit in improving menopausal symptoms such as hot flashes, night sweats, nervousness, headaches, heart palpitations, and the buildup of the vaginal lining. However, another study showed that black cohosh did not help with hot flashes.[11]

Unfortunately, these clinical studies were very small, evaluating only sixty to eighty-five women and were very short, lasting only two to six months. This is not long enough to determine the long-term safety of black cohosh. It took the Women's Health Initiative study five years looking at over sixteen thousand women to be able to determine the long-term risks and benefits of estrogen. The shorter studies are limited because menopausal symptoms have a significant placebo response that does not start to diminish until after three months. So even though there is scant evidence that black cohosh may be helpful with menopausal symptoms, it is still unclear if it is safe to take. Some of the long-term concerns with black cohosh and other remedies will be detailed later.

*Evening Primrose (*Oenothera biennis*)*

Oil of evening primrose (also known as evening star) is rich in gamma-linolenic acid, a type of omega-3 essential fatty acid. A single, well-done clinical trial exists on the effect of primrose oil on menopause. This study, a six-month randomized, double-blind, placebo-controlled study of fifty-six women comparing evening primrose oil (EPO) at 2,000 mg and vitamin E at 20 mg twice a day, showed no benefit from either for the treatment of hot flashes.[12]

Evening primrose oil is also commonly recommended for breast pain and PMS. There is some evidence that evening primrose oil can help with breast pain but it can take months to take effect.[13] Most of the studies looking at evening primrose oil and PMS shows no improvement over placebo.[14] Evening primrose oil does contain several anticoagulant substances. These substances may decrease the blood's ability to clot, potentially leading to bleeding problems if taken in high enough doses, and should be avoided especially in women who are taking anticoagulants or other blood thinners.

*Dong Quai (*Angelica sinensis*)*

Dong Quai is a root of a type of angelica used in traditional Chinese medicine for a number of gynecological problems. Dong Quai supposedly regulates and balances the menstrual cycle and strengthens the uterus.[15] The limited studies available have not shown Dong Quai to have any improvement over placebo in the treatment of hot flashes. Some critics argue that Dong Quai is usually added to other botanical products for its effect, but most women who purchase it do not get it from a traditional Chinese medicine herbalist and use it alone. Moreover, the cumulative effect of all these untested herbs could pose a health risk.

Dong Quai contains coumarins which are anticoagulants that can interfere with the clotting of blood. There is also some conflicting data showing that Dong Quai may stimulate breast cancer cells.[16] Other substances in Dong Quai such as safrole and psoralen are carcinogenic.[17] Given the lack of documented efficacy and the number of potentially serious problems it may trigger, Dong Quai should be avoided for the treatment of menopausal symptoms.

Red Clover *(*Trifolium pratense*)*

Red clover is a rich source of a number of isoflavones, a phytoestrogen that is a plant compound that acts like estrogens. Two studies looking at the effectiveness of red clover on menopausal symptoms showed no difference from placebo for the treatment of hot flashes.[18] Of interest in one study was that the more isoflavones in the woman's urine, the fewer hot flashes she had whether in the treated or placebo group. This may indicate that women who naturally have a diet high in isoflavones (soy being the most common source) and/or who absorb isoflavones well when eaten, may have fewer hot flashes.

Isoflavones may also be helpful in preventing osteoporosis, though this data is mixed. No adverse effects were seen in any of the studies, but the longest study was for *only six months*. Some concern exists as to the presence of coumarins in red clover extracts, which is an anticoagulant (and may affect the clotting ability of blood). Other concerns include the effects of the iso-flavones on the uterus and breast. Though some studies have shown no stimu-latory effect on the lining of the uterus, the studies, again, were only for six months. Because isoflavones may act on estrogen receptors, there is some con-cern that long-term use of isoflavones such as red clover may increase the risk of breast and uterine cancer, though there is no data to show this at this time.[19]

Wild Yam Creams

Wild yam contains diosgenin, a plant compound that is chemically altered to form hormones. Some wild yam creams seemed to help some women with their menopausal symptoms, which fueled an interest in wild yam creams. However, testing by independent labs found several yam creams adulterated with progesterone and even estrogen.[20] If a woman used one of these products, she may have noticed an improvement in her menopausal symptoms because both estrogen and progesterone have been shown to help with menopausal symptoms.[21] Unfortunately, these women would have unknowingly been on hormones and could have had serious problems induced by them without realizing it.

The human body does not have the enzymes to convert the diosgenin found in wild yams into hormones in the body. So although the diosgenin has been used to synthesize hormones through a chemical process, it has not been found to be more effective than placebo for hot flashes.

Ginseng

A wide variety of ginseng products come under the label of ginseng: American ginseng, Chinese or Korean ginseng, and Siberian ginseng. The different types of ginseng may work differently so you cannot assume that they will have the same effect. Ginseng is touted for boosting immunity and energy, and may have some estrogen-like effects as well. One sixteen-week study with 384 women showed that a ginseng product had no better effect than placebo for hot flashes. However, it did show some improvement for depression, general health, and well-being.[22] However, we're talking of a study over only four months.

One of the main problems with studying ginseng is the variety of ginseng products on the market. Another barrier is the extremely wide variations in the amount of active ingredients and the addition of large amounts of caffeine in several of the preparations. One study found that only one in four of the products touting ginseng actually contained it.[23]

Additional concerns are the estrogen-like activity of ginseng. Uterine bleeding has occurred after ginseng use. Although one study did not show any effect on the endometrium (the lining of the uterus), the study again was only sixteen weeks long.[24] Some evidence shows that ginseng may induce the growth of breast cancer cells.[25]

Other side effects include high blood pressure, insomnia, headache, irritability, diarrhea, nausea, breast tenderness, and palpitations.[26] It is unclear how much of this is due to ginseng or the other compounds added to the ginseng that may not be listed on the label. Ginseng may also interact with other medicines, either increasing or decreasing their levels in the body. Ginseng should be avoided in people with cardiovascular disease, high blood pressure, and diabetes and should be taken with caution with other medications.

Chasteberry (Chaste Tree; **Vitex agnus-castus***)*

Chasteberry is a dried ripe fruit of the chaste tree that was used in ancient Greece. Chasteberry contains hormonelike substances and has been recommended for hot flashes, breast tenderness, and PMS. Although there are no clinical studies showing that chasteberry helps hot flashes, one study showed that it was more effective than placebo over three cycles in reducing PMS symptoms of irritability, breast fullness, and bloating.[27] However, other studies have not confirmed this finding.[28]

Side effects of chasteberry include gastrointestinal complaints, itching, rash, headaches, fatigue, and hair loss. Beyond three menstrual cycles, we have no idea what additional symptoms or problems may arise. It may also interact with certain medications such as birth control pills.[29]

Licorice *(Glycyrrhiza glabra)*

Licorice supposedly has estrogenlike activity. Most licorice sold as candy in the United States is actually anise-flavored sugar and not licorice. To date, no clinical studies have examined its effectiveness for treating menopausal symptoms. Licorice has been associated with high blood pressure, fluid retention, and preterm birth.

Flaxseed Oil *(Linum usitatissimum; Linseed oil)*

Flaxseed oil, also known as linseed oil, contains high concentrations of lignans, a phytoestrogen. Very few studies have been done on the effect of flaxseed oil in the treatment of menopausal symptoms. The data have been mixed. This could be due to the variety of ways flaxseed can be given, which include ground whole flaxseed baked in breads, oils used in foods, and concentrated tablets containing flaxseed extracts.

Flaxseed is a rich source of the omega-3 fatty acid. Because of this, it may have a beneficial effect on cholesterol levels and reduce the risk of heart disease. Some studies show some improvement in the cholesterol levels of women taking flaxseed oil.[30] Supplementing your diet with foods made with flaxseed oil is one thing, but the side effects and long-term effects of taking large amounts of concentrated flaxseed oil remain unknown at this time.

Soy

Soy has generated great interest as an alternative to estrogen in treating menopausal symptoms. Soy contains phytoestrogens, which are plant compounds that may act like estrogens in the human body. Populations with diets containing large amounts of phytoestrogens have fewer hot flashes. Fewer than 25 percent of Japanese and Chinese women complain of hot flashes compared to 75 to 85 percent of women in North America and Europe.[31] Asian women also have less cardiovascular disease, osteoporosis, breast, endometrial, ovarian, and colon cancer.[32]

Is the reason for this difference related to a diet high in phytoestrogens?

Or could it be related to other factors such as cultural differences, other aspects of their diet, physical activity, or some as-yet-unidentified factor? Even if the differences are found to be related to phytoestrogen in the diet, it may be a lifetime of increased intake that causes the difference. In other words, starting a diet high in phytoestrogens during perimenopause may not provide the benefits seen in these other populations. It is also unclear if taking megadoses of phytoestrogens is safe.

The studies looking into the effect of soy on hot flashes have been mixed. Part of the problem is the wide range of soy products used in the studies; soy beverages, high-soy diets; different types of soy proteins; or tablets or capsules containing soy extracts, isolated isoflavones (a type of phytoestrogen), or a mixture of the two. Amounts of soy and isoflavones also differed from study to study.[33] The studies may also be affected by the variability of phytoestrogen content in food.[34] Studies on the effect of soy on bone density, cholesterol, and blood pressure are also inconclusive.

Soy foods have been a regular part of the Asian diet for thousands of years and do not seem to cause health problems when taken as part of a normal Asian diet. Soy foods provide a good source of protein. However, the safety of soy in doses significantly greater than that taken in the typical Asian diet is unknown. While the relatively lower levels of phytoestrogens taken naturally in the diet may be beneficial to one's health, you cannot assume that more phytoestrogen will increase the benefit. More phytoestrogen may actually have the opposite effect.

And this is where the big question lies. In cases where phytoestrogen or another herbal product helps with hot flashes and other menopausal problems by acting like an estrogen, couldn't they also have the same problems that prescribed estrogens have? The answer is still unclear.

Some women with breast cancer, who were advised against taking estrogen for fear of increasing the chance of recurrence of the disease, turned to alternatives to help with their menopausal symptoms. They may have turned to "natural remedies" such as soy extracts or other herbal treatments thinking them to be safer. Unfortunately, it is unknown if they are safer or not: since they may have an estrogen-like effect on cancer, they could possibly increase the risk of recurrence. The American College of Obstetricians and Gynecologists warns in regard to soy and isoflavones: "Given the possibility that these compounds may interact with estrogen, these agents should not be considered free of potential harm in women with estrogen-dependent cancers."[35]

BOTANICAL OR HERBAL REMEDIES FOR OTHER SYMPTOMS

St. John's Wort (Hypericum perforatum)

Extracts of this flower have been used for centuries to treat mild to moderate depression. In Germany, it is licensed for the treatment of anxiety, depression, and sleep disorders. St. John's wort contains at least ten compounds that may contribute to its effect. How it works is still unclear.

A number of studies have shown that St. John's wort is more effective than placebo in treating mild to moderate depression and is similar in effectiveness to low doses of tricyclic antidepressants.[36] Tricyclic antidepressants are an older medication for depression. St. John's wort may help with depressive symptoms related to menopause.

St. John's wort has some side effects, the most prominent being photosensitivity.[37] Photosensitivity occurs when a substance gets into the skin and makes it react differently to sunlight. It can cause the skin to burn, form a rash, or itch. Other symptoms include dry mouth, dizziness, constipation, and nausea.[38]

Of more concern, St. John's wort has been shown to interact with other medications and may decrease the blood levels of a large range of prescribed medications such as birth control pills, reducing their effectiveness. Using St John's wort with a class of antidepressants called selective serotonin reuptake inhibitors (including Prozac, Paxil, Zoloft, Effexor, and Celexa) can lead to serotonin overload, and thus can pose a danger.[39]

Because of the possibility of its interaction with other medications, St. John's wort should not be used with other antidepressants and only very cautiously with other medications. Before you do take St. John's wort, you should confer with your physician to see how it may affect the other medications you may be taking. Unfortunately, there is very little data on the effect of St. John's wort on specific medications.

Valerian Root (Valeriana officinalis)

Valerian root has been used for over a thousand years to help decrease anxiety and stress and to improve sleep. Insomnia and other sleep disorders become more common during perimenopause and menopause, so some women have turned to valerian root for help. The active ingredient is still unknown. To date, studies have shown mixed results in its effectiveness for the treatment of sleep disorders.

Side effects include headache and morning grogginess. Little is known about its interactions with other drugs. Because of its potential sedative effect, valerian should never be mixed with alcohol and other sedatives.[40]

Kava (Piper methysticum)

Kava is a shrub grown throughout the Pacific islands and has been used to reduce anxiety and relieve pain. A small eight-week study in postmenopausal women showed that it helped decrease anxiety and hot flashes over placebo.[41] Several other small studies have also shown kava to help with anxiety.[42] Again, these were small studies over a very short period.

Kava may affect your ability to drive, may cause skin reactions, and may upset your stomach. Kava should not be used with alcohol or other sedatives. Unfortunately, kava has also been associated with liver failure, which should give you pause.[43] As noted above, the sale of kava has been banned in Canada, Singapore, the United Kingdom, and other European nations.

VITAMINS AND MINERALS

Many women are now turning to vitamins and minerals as a "safe" alternative to medications. The ideal way to get these key nutrients is through your diet. Fresh fruits and vegetables are an excellent source of vitamins and also provide other benefits such as fiber and other nutrients that may be beneficial to your health.

Taking megadoses of vitamins have not been shown to improve health and may be harmful. High doses of certain vitamins such as the fat soluble vitamins (vitamins A, D, E, and K) as well as B6 can may be toxic. Taking a general multivitamin would be reasonable to ensure that you are getting enough vitamins without overdoing it.

Vitamin E

Vitamin E has been recognized as a potent antioxidant. Major sources of vitamin E include salad oils, margarine, nuts, and legumes. It may help lower cholesterol and insulin levels and possibly decrease the risk of cardiovascular disease.[44] Vitamin E has also been used for the treatment of hot flashes. However, a recent placebo-controlled study looked at vitamin E

400 IU taken twice daily and found marginal benefit over placebo (one less hot flash per day over placebo).[45]

Vitamin E was thought to be effective for PMS for many years. Studies in the 1980s suggested a benefit, but later studies failed to confirm this.[46] At this time, there is no strong evidence showing vitamin E to be helpful for PMS.

Vitamin E in doses from 200 to 800 mg (IU) per day is generally well tolerated, though some people get upset stomach. Doses from 800 to 1,200 mg per day may cause bleeding problems because of the effect of vitamin E on platelets. Above 1,200 mg per day can result in headache, fatigue, nausea, diarrhea, cramping, weakness, blurry vision, and possibly worse.[47]

Folate (Folic Acid)

Folate is a B vitamin that is found in high concentrations in dark-green leafy vegetables and whole-grain cereals. Taking more folate may decrease the risk of heart disease and stroke.[48] Vitamins B6 and B12 may also play a role in decreasing the risk of coronary heart disease.

There is also some evidence that folate may decrease the risk of breast and colon cancers. It is unclear whether taking extra folate is beneficial for all women or only for those women who have low folate levels.[49] It also decreases the risk of neural tube defects (a birth defect where there is an opening over the spinal cord or brain) in babies as they grow inside of pregnant women. Folate seems to be well tolerated with rare side effects. The main concern is that taking doses above 1,000 mg per day may mask a certain type of anemia caused by a vitamin B12 deficiency.

A dose of 400 to 800 micrograms of folate along with 3 micrograms of vitamin B6 and 9 micrograms of vitamin B12 found in most general multivitamins would be a reasonable amount to take until further information becomes available.

Vitamin B6

Vitamin B6 refers to a group of compounds that are found in poultry, fish, meat, legumes, nuts, potatoes, and whole grains. Marginal vitamin B6 intake may increase the risk of heart disease.[50]

Vitamin B6 may be one of the most commonly used supplements for PMS. However, the studies done to date have been generally of poor quality, which limits their conclusions. The results suggest some benefit for mood symptoms as well as breast tenderness, nonetheless.[51] Neurotoxicity can be seen when higher doses are taken and vitamin B6 should be limited to 100 mg per day.[52]

Vitamin D (Calciferol)

Vitamin D helps you absorb calcium from the intestines. Vitamin D is made when your body is exposed to the sun. Vitamin D is also found in fortified milk, saltwater fish, and fish-liver oil. Fifteen minutes in the sun a day is all you need to produce the vitamin D you require. As you get older, your body's ability to make vitamin D decreases.

Inadequate levels of vitamin D is more common than people realize, especially among the elderly and those with little exposure to sunlight. Vitamin D with calcium has been shown to decrease bone loss and fracture rates in the elderly. Women over age sixty-five should take 400 to 800 IU of vitamin D to help with calcium absorption.

Vitamin C (Ascorbic Acid)

Vitamin C is a strong antioxidant found in citrus fruits, strawberries, melons, tomatoes, broccoli, and peppers. Vitamin C does not seem to have a large impact on the risk of cardiovascular disease. Diets high in vitamin C are associated with a decreased risk of breast, stomach, esophagus, and oral cancers, though the source of vitamin C in most of these studies was from high fruit and vegetable intake.[53] It is unclear if the benefit is related to vitamin C or the high intake of fruits and vegetables, which provide a wide range of other nutrients that may also affect the cancer risk. No studies have shown that extra vitamin C by itself decreases the risk of cancer.

The current recommended daily intake of vitamin C is 60 mg per day. Doses up to 1,500 mg are well tolerated. Higher doses can be associated with nausea and diarrhea.[54]

Magnesium

Magnesium is a mineral that may also play a role in bone health. A deficiency of magnesium may lead to bone loss.[55] About two-thirds of the body's magnesium is contained in the skeleton.[56] Magnesium is found in dark green vegetables, soy products, most nuts, seeds, legumes, and whole grains.

There is also evidence that a deficiency of magnesium may also be associated with an increased risk of cardiovascular disease, high blood pressure, and diabetes.[57] Whether taking extra magnesium will help prevent these diseases is still unclear.

Reduced levels of magnesium have been reported in women with PMS. A small study showed magnesium reduced PMS symptoms. Women took magnesium pyrrolidone carboxylic acid containing 360 mg of magnesium three times a day starting on the fifteenth day of the menstrual cycle until the first day of bleeding.[58]

This was a small study of only thirty-two women, so more data is needed to confirm that magnesium is truly effective for the treatment of PMS. Another small study showed magnesium pyrrolidone carboxylic acid to decrease menstrual migraine headaches.[59] Possible side effects of magnesium include bloating, cramping, and diarrhea.

Once again, megadoses of any vitamins or mineral can be dangerous and should be taken only under the advice and supervision of your physician.

OTHER ALTERNATIVE THERAPIES

Homeopathy

Homeopathy is a system of medicine originated by Samuel Hahnemann in 1796 based on the principle of "like cures like." Different substances were tested on healthy people and their symptoms were recorded. These substances were then diluted over and over again. The more dilute the substance, the more potent it supposedly became. This sounds counterintuitive but the theory is that the dilution process is what increases the strength of the homeopathic medicine.

If someone developed a symptom, the substance that caused the symptom in the healthy person was given in very dilute doses to the person that was ill. The reasoning thus went: the substance that caused the symptom at full dose would be used in very dilute amounts to cure that same symptom. This approach is more popular in Europe, but has been gaining popularity here.

There remains still much debate as to whether homeopathy is effective medical therapy. At this time, there are no homeopathic remedies that have been proven to be more effective than placebo in the treatment of menopausal symptoms.

Acupuncture

Acupuncture has been a part of traditional Chinese medicine for thousands of years. Acupuncture is based on the principle that there is movement of energy called "qi" in the body along channels called meridians. Adherents believe that when this energy is excessive, deficient, blocked, or misdirected, it can upset the balance in the body and lead to illness. Needles are placed along the meridians to return the natural flow of energy.

Few side effects have been seen as a result of acupuncture, with the main concern being the use of reusable needles which may lead to infections or blood-borne viruses. Most acupuncturists in the United States use disposable needles because of this fear.

According to a National Institutes of Health consensus panel of scientists, researchers, and practitioners who met in November 1997, clinical studies have shown that acupuncture is effective in the treatment of post-operative nausea, and vomiting and dental pain after surgery.[60] Acupuncture may be useful to treat a number of other conditions. No studies have yet shown acupuncture to be useful in the treatment of menopausal symptoms.[61] One study comparing electroacupuncture to a control group who had shallow acupuncture needles insertion at the same point showed no difference in hot flashes or sleep.[62]

T'ai Chi

T'ai Chi has been described as a form of exercise, a martial art, as meditation, and as a part of traditional Chinese medicine. Adherents believe that its slow circular movements help the flow of energy or "qi" through the body. Studies have shown T'ai Chi to improve balance and reduce falls in the elderly, but so have other studies on exercise.[63] T'ai Chi's effect on menopausal symptoms is still unknown.

Aruveda

Aruvedic medicine is the oldest medical system known, originating in India. The principle behind aruvedic medicine is that imbalances among the three basic bodily humors can lead to disease. Diet, massage, vomiting, enemas, and meditation are used to heal the body. There is little data about its use for menopausal symptoms, though meditation and relaxation may be useful for stress reduction.[64]

Yoga

Yoga is a practice that involves the use of breathing exercises, physical postures, and meditation. It complements aruvedic medicine. Yoga has been shown to reduce stress, blood pressure, and improve physical fitness.

Little data exist about the use of aruvedic medicine or yoga for menopausal symptoms. The meditation may promote stress reduction, which may help with some menopausal symptoms.

Naturopathy

Naturopathy uses a combination of herbs, dietary changes, massage, and relaxation therapies to treat medical problems. Naturopathy may use any alternative or complementary practices in addition to traditional medicine to heal the body. The relaxation therapies may also promote stress reduction. (Please refer to the section on dietary supplements above for more information on herbal remedies and their use during menopause.)

Aromatherapy

Aromatherapy uses smells, both pleasant and unpleasant, obtained from the oils of aromatic plants for the purpose of enhancing health and beauty. No studies have shown that aromatherapy enhances beauty or helps with menopausal symptoms, but it may help with relaxation.

Biofeedback

Biofeedback uses monitors to provide feedback on different parts of your body. Biofeedback has been used successfully to improve symptoms of incontinence, anxiety, headaches, and muscle pain.[65] It has not been used for menopausal symptoms, but biofeedback may be a useful tool in the treatment of some of these other problems that are more common in perimenopausal and menopausal women, although there is no data on its use in this group of women.

Chiropractic Medicine

Adherents of chiropractic medicine believe that spinal manipulation and adjustment treat a number of conditions, usually back and neck problems and headaches. It has not been shown to help with alleviating menopausal symptoms.[66]

Massage

Massage or other body-touching therapies have been used throughout the ages. Your skin is the largest organ in your body. Human touch is vital to growth and health. This is most poignantly demonstrated in institutionalized children who have had all of their physical needs met, but still fail to grow and thrive. Though no studies have researched the effect of massage on menopausal symptoms, it does help with relaxation. When oils are used, some people can have a reaction to them. But overall, most people enjoy a massage if only for the short-term pleasure and relaxation it provides.

Relaxation and Meditation

A number of different techniques to help with relaxation and meditation are available. Meditation has been shown to help reduce stress, panic, anxiety, and pain. It has also been shown to reduce muscle tension and decrease blood pressure. Hot flashes cause a reaction similar to a stress response and it has been thought that relaxation techniques may therefore help reduce hot flashes.[67]

Several small studies have looked at various relaxation methods and their effect on hot flashes. One study using diaphragmatic breathing as the mental focus showed a decrease in the intensity of hot flashes, but not in the number. It also showed a decrease in anxiety, tension, and depression.[68] Two other small studies found a decrease in hot flashes with different breathing and muscle relaxation exercises.[69] Even if relaxation and meditation have no effect on menopausal symptoms, they have no known adverse effects and are free, and therefore using them to decrease stress may be beneficial in general and is a reasonable option to improve your overall health.

Exercise

Exercise has many health benefits including reducing the risk of heart disease, diabetes, and osteoporosis, and improving mood, strength, and balance. Exercise may even help with hot flashes. One survey showed that women who exercised three or more times a week had fewer hot flashes.[70] Even if it doesn't work for everyone, the overwhelming health benefits of regular exercise cannot be ignored and should be a regular part of your daily life.

Magnets

Magnets have been gaining popularity in the treatment of various types of pain. Few randomized double-blind, placebo-controlled studies have been done to date. Some studies show that they do help and other studies show no improvement over placebo.[71] The problem with studies on magnet therapy are the different types and strengths of magnets and that most people can quickly figure out if they are in the magnet or placebo arm of the study.

A single small study looked at magnets in the treatment of hot flashes and showed no decrease of hot flashes over placebo.[72]

Vaginal Lubricants

Vaginal dryness is not an uncommon complaint as women get older and go through menopause. Estrogen is important in producing lubrication when a woman becomes aroused. With the drop in estrogen that accompanies menopause, women notice a decrease in quality and quantity of lubrication. Over-the-counter lubricants are available. Water-based lubricants, such as Astroglide and KY Jelly, are the best. (See chapter 6.)

THE BOTTOM LINE

There are a number of alternatives available that are being promoted to help with perimenopausal and menopausal symptoms. Many of these alternatives have not been rigorously studied and may derive much if not all of their supposed benefit from the placebo response. Some of these alternatives are good for your overall health such as exercise and relaxation techniques. However, other remedies may be of little benefit and may pose significant unknown health risks. Caveat emptor. Let the buyer beware has never been so true.

CHAPTER 11

LIFE AFTER MENOPAUSE

Menopause is kind of sad. But there's a good side: The children are all grown. We now have our own time for ourselves to enjoy our life.

—Lily Kim

Finally, you've made it through menopause. No more periods. Many of your symptoms are probably improved or resolved. Some women rejoice while others may feel a bit sad and nostalgic because they have passed another stage of their lives. At this time, certain issues such as contraception and hormonal fluctuations are no longer a concern. However, other problems come to the forefront such as osteoporosis, heart disease, and stroke, which are major causes of disability and death in women. The likelihood of these diseases increases with age.

OSTEOPOROSIS

Osteoporosis is a progressive disease in which the bone gets so thin that it can break with little or no trauma. Picking up a heavy object, sitting too hard, or even coughing can lead to a fracture when bones become this fragile. As you are growing, your bones get stronger and thicker, especially

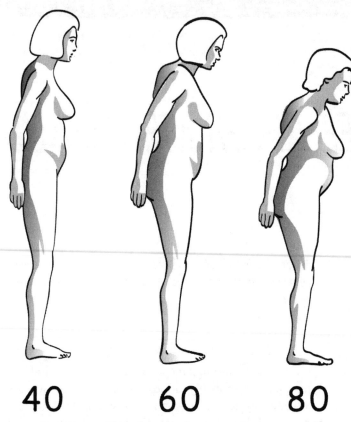

40   60   80

Figure 11.1. *The effects of osteoporosis.*

during puberty. Your bones are the strongest and thickest when you are in your twenties.[1] After that time, your bones gradually thin until menopause, at which time there is an acceleration of bone loss due to declining estrogen levels.[2] The accelerated loss occurs in the first ten to fifteen years after menopause, after which time it slows but continues at a lesser rate.[3]

Many people think of bones as dried up dead tissue that doesn't change once you've reached your adult height. However, your bones are a living, dynamic structure made up of collagen fibers on which calcium is deposited to give bones their strength. Your bones are constantly changing and remodeling. Old bone is broken down, removed, and replaced by new bone. This helps keep your bones strong, strengthening them in areas in response to stress. Hormones, exercise, and calcium intake are some of the factors that help maintain strength in your bones.

During the first twenty to thirty years of your life, you build up bone faster than you break it down. This makes your bones thicker, denser, and stronger. After that time, bone is broken down faster than it is built up, leading to a gradual weakening of your bones; this increases further after menopause. When your bones become very thin, either from losing too much bone, not building enough bone, or a combination of the two, osteoporosis is the result.

Osteoporosis: The Effects

Osteoporosis threatens forty-four million Americans. Thirty-four million have low-bone mass and ten million already have osteoporosis.[4] Of the people with osteoporosis, eight out of ten are women, making it much more common in women. Half of all women will have an osteoporosis-related fracture in their lifetime. There are 1.5 million osteoporotic fractures a year with 700,000 vertebral fractures, 250,000 distal forearm fractures, 250,000 hip fractures, and 300,000 fractures of other sites.[5] Besides the initial cost of treating and caring for these patients, many of these women will go on to develop chronic pain and long-term disabilities that will limit their ability to care for themselves.

Osteoporosis: The Cost

Hip fractures are one of the most serious complications of osteoporosis. Up to 20 percent of women die in the first six months after fracturing their hip. Another 50 percent will be unable to walk or perform activities of daily living without assistance and 25 percent will require long-term care.[6]

Other common osteoporotic fracture sites besides the hip include the spine, arm, and wrist. Many women with osteoporosis suffer from vertebral compression fractures. The spine is made up of bones called vertebrae that are stacked on top of each other like blocks. As the bones get thinner, the vertebrae weaken and the weight of the spine on the vertebrae causes them to collapse. Initially there is intense pain that lasts for two to three weeks and then usually gradually subsides over the next three to four months. However, the pain may evolve into a chronic condition limiting a woman's ability to function.[7]

Dowager's hump—(the hump on the upper back that forms in some older women that makes them look hunched over) which is what most people associate with osteoporosis—is the result of multiple compression fractures of the thoracic or middle part of the spine.

Risk Factors for Osteoporosis

A number of risk factors may put you at increased risk for osteoporosis, including:

- Gender: women are much more likely to develop osteoporosis than men
- Age: your bones become thinner as you age, increasing the risk of osteoporosis
- Body size: being thin increases the risk of osteoporosis, especially if you are less than 127 pounds
- Ethnicity: Caucasian and Asian women are at higher risk, but all women are at risk
- Family history: if your parents have osteoporosis, you have a higher risk of getting osteoporosis
- Personal history of fracture after age fifty
- Smoking: yet another reason to stop smoking
- Early menopause: if you had both your ovaries removed or went through menopause before forty-five, this increases your risk for osteoporosis
- Lifelong diet low in calcium: your bones are made up mostly of calcium and you need to take it to strengthen your bones
- Alcoholism: another reason to cut back on alcohol
- Anorexia: anorexia leads to low estrogen levels, which decreases the ability of the bone to build up, especially during the critical teens and twenties when the bones are growing
- Sedentary lifestyle: walking and other weight-bearing activities help to strengthen your bones
- Medications: certain medications such as steroids, heparin, and anti-seizure medications increase the risk of osteoporosis
- Medical illnesses: Conditions such as hyperthyroidism, hyperparathyroidism, Cushing's disease, and diabetes increase the risk of osteoporosis

Prevention of Osteoporosis

Some of these risk factors, such as your gender, age, ethnicity, and family history, can't be changed. Neither can a life of poor calcium intake or past history of anorexia. But you can address some of these other factors to help decrease your risk of getting osteoporosis. We will look at these factors in depth, but first, if you have children, you can do a lot to help them develop stronger bones.

Help Your Children Develop Strong Bones

Since most of the bone is built up during adolescence, some people contend that osteoporosis is a disease of adolescence that doesn't show up until after menopause. Think of your skeleton as a storage place, or bank, for bone. You store the most bone when you are young, especially in your teens, and the amount you store during that time is what you have to use the rest of your life. To help your adolescent children build up their "bone bank," make sure they get enough calcium, 1,300 mg a day. That's over a quart of milk a day, every day. If they are not milk drinkers, they can drink calcium-fortified drinks or take a calcium supplement. Regular activity is also important to build up their bones. These two steps will help immensely with their future bone health and may help prevent osteoporosis in their distant future.

Now back to you.

Smoking and Alcohol Can Hurt Bones

Smoking and excess alcohol use are associated with a number of health problems, including osteoporosis. Excess alcohol use not only increases the risk of osteoporosis, but it also increases the risk for falls or injuries that may lead to the breaking of your weakened bones.

Exercise Strengthens Bones

Weight-bearing activities—where your body supports its own weight, as opposed to swimming where the water supports your weight—help keep your bones strong. These include walking, aerobics, and stairsteppers. The stress of your weight on the bones causes them to remodel and build up the areas of stress, strengthening the bones overall. Physical activity also strengthens your muscles and improves balance so that you are less likely to fall and less likely to break a bone even if your bones are weaker.

Calcium, the Building Blocks of Bone

Your bones hold your body's main reservoir of calcium. Calcium is vital to the functioning of the cells in your body, including the contracting of your muscles, the regulation of your heartbeat, and the proper functioning of your nerves. Calcium must be maintained within certain levels or serious problems can result. If your intake of calcium is inadequate, your body draws the calcium from your bones to maintain this level of calcium in the rest of your body.

An adequate intake of calcium is vital to keep your bones strong and to keep your body from taking the calcium from your bones in order to function. As you get older, you absorb less calcium from your intestines and release more calcium through your kidneys. However, taking calcium alone cannot reverse bone loss or treat osteoporosis once the damage has been done. The following table is a guideline for how much calcium you should take a day.

Recommended Calcium Intake

Age	Daily Calcium Intake (mg per day)
Birth to 6 months	210
6 to 12 months	270
1 to 3 years	500
4 to 8 years	800
9 to 18 years	1300
19 to 50 years	1000
51 and older	1200

How Do You Get Enough Calcium?

Calcium is found in many foods. Dairy products are the most common foods that people associate with calcium and they do contain a lot of calcium. Here are some examples of foods and their calcium content (generally the low-fat version of the food such as milk does not change its calcium content):

Food	Amount	Calcium (mg)
Milk (whole, 2%, skim)	1 cup	300
Yogurt	1 cup	300
Ice cream	½ cup	100
Cottage cheese	½ cup	100
Cheddar cheese	1 oz.	110
Broccoli	½ cup	40
Orange	1 medium	50
Banana	1 medium	10
Bread (white and whole wheat)	1 slice	25
Beef (roasted)	3 oz.	7
Chicken (roasted)	3 oz.	13
Beans (kidney, navy, pinto)	1 cup	90
Tofu	½ cup	130
Salmon, with bones (canned)	3 oz.	200

For foods with labels, look at the calcium content which is listed as a percentage. Multiply the percentage by 10 and you will have the number of milligrams of calcium in a serving. For example, if a label states that a serving contains 20 percent calcium, you would multiply that by 10 and get 200, which would be the number of milligrams of calcium in a serving.

For many women, getting the necessary amount of calcium is difficult. Dairy products contain a significant amount of calcium, but unfortunately many people become lactose intolerant as they get older. Lactose is the main sugar in milk. An enzyme breaks down the lactose in the small intestine so it can be absorbed by the body. Some people produce inadequate amounts of this enzyme so that when they consume dairy products, they may develop nausea, cramping, bloating, gas, and diarrhea a half hour to two hours later. Lactose-free dairy products are available, as are other calcium-enriched foods such as calcium-fortified orange juice. Even so, it may be difficult to take in 1,000 mg or more of calcium every day through diet alone.

Calcium Supplements

Women can turn to calcium supplements to get the correct amount of calcium. There are an enormous number of choices for calcium supplementation. Different types of calcium compounds include calcium carbonate, calcium citrate, and calcium phosphate. Calcium can also come in pills, liquids, powders, candies, and chewable forms. They can also be found in a wide range of strengths. With all these choices, it can become very confusing when deciding which one to pick.

Which calcium supplement is the best? There is no "best" calcium supplement. The best one for you may not be well tolerated by someone else. Some women have trouble swallowing pills. For them, a liquid, powder, or chewable form may be the best.

Types of Calcium Supplements

Calcium carbonate, calcium citrate, and calcium phosphate are different calcium compounds that are all good sources of calcium. Some women will have side effects, such as bloating, stomach upset, or constipation, from one form and not on another. Changing the form of the calcium from a pill to a chewable form may also help with side effects. When choosing a calcium supplement, it is important to look at the actual amount of calcium in each tablet. For example, regular strength TUMS is a 500 mg tablet, but contains 200 mg of calcium.

You generally want to choose a calcium supplement from a reliable source such as a brand name with proven reliability and/or one with the USP (United States Pharmacopeia) symbol. The United States Pharmacopeia is a nongovernment organization that protects the public health by establishing state-of-the-art standards to ensure the quality of medicines and other health care technologies. Having the USP symbol indicates that the product meets their standards for purity and quality. Because seeking this approval is voluntary, there may be good products without this symbol, but you cannot be sure. If the calcium comes from unrefined oyster shell, bone meal, or dolomite, you will want to be certain the bottle has the USP symbol, because those without may have higher levels of lead and other toxic metals.

When to Take Calcium

Generally, it is best to take the calcium supplement with meals because the acid produced by your stomach when eating helps with absorbing the calcium. Your body has a hard time absorbing more than 500 mg of calcium at a time, whether it is in the food or a tablet, so it is best to space out your calcium intake throughout the day. If you drink a large glass of milk at breakfast, it would be better to take the calcium supplement with a different meal. Calcium can also diminish the absorption of other medications. If you take any other medications, you will want to check to see if you need to avoid taking it with your calcium.

Many women are concerned that calcium supplements may increase the risk of kidney stones since they are usually made out of calcium. The data on this is mixed and if you have a history of kidney stones, you should seek advice from your physician before starting on calcium supplements at all.[8]

Magnesium

Magnesium is a mineral that may also play a role in bone health. A deficiency of magnesium may lead to bone loss.[9] About two-thirds of the body's magnesium is contained in the skeleton. Magnesium is found in dark green vegetables, soy products, most nuts, seeds, legumes (such as beans and peas), and whole grains. According to the U.S. Department of Agriculture Research Service, the best ratio of calcium to magnesium is 2 to 1. In other words, if 1,000 mg of calcium is taken in, about 500 mg of magnesium should also be taken. There is also evidence that a deficiency of magnesium may also be associated with an increased risk of cardiovascular disease, high blood pressure, and diabetes. It is still unclear whether magnesium supplements will help prevent these diseases.[10]

Vitamin D

Vitamin D helps you absorb calcium from the intestines. Vitamin D is made when your body is exposed to the sun. Fifteen minutes in the sun a day is all you need to produce the vitamin D you need. As you get older, your body's ability to make vitamin D decreases. Women over age sixty-five should take 400 to 800 IU of vitamin D to help with calcium absorption.

Diagnosing Osteoporosis

How can you tell if you have osteoporosis? Osteoporosis is like high cholesterol: you don't have any symptoms until it causes a major problem like a heart attack. Similarly, osteoporosis is a silent disease until it causes a fracture, but by then it's too late to do much about it. Bone density testing is the best test to determine the strength of the bones.

There are several ways that bone density can be determined:

- DEXA (Dual Energy X-Ray Absorptiometry) measures the hip, spine, or total body
- pDXA (Peripheral Dual Energy X-Ray Absorptiometry) measures the wrist, heel, or finger
- QCT (Quantitative Computerized Tomography) measures the hip, spine, or total body
- Ultrasonometry measures the heel, shinbone, or kneecap

DEXA, pDXA, and QCT use very small amounts of X-rays to scan your bones. Ultrasonometry uses ultrasound. These tests take up to fifteen minutes to perform and are painless. The amount of radiation used is very low, less than a dental X-ray. The density of your bones is compared to the bone density of a healthy young adult and given a score called the T-score. A T-score above –1.0 is normal. A T-score of –1.0 to –2.5 is called osteopenia, which means that your bones are significantly thinner than normal. A T-score of less than –2.5 is osteoporosis.

Who Should Have Bone Density Testing?

There is still some controversy as to who needs to have this screening test, but most experts now recommend that all women sixty-five and older be screened. Because of the large numbers of women who will develop osteoporosis, many physicians advocate that all postmenopausal women be screened since risk factors for osteoporosis do not accurately predict who will have fractures.

The National Osteoporosis Foundation suggests the following people have bone density screening:[11]

- All women sixty-five or older
- Women under age sixty-five with one or more additional risk factors for osteoporosis besides menopause (see risk factors above)
- A postmenopausal woman who has just had a fracture
- A woman who is considering therapy for osteoporosis, if bone density testing will help her make a final decision
- A woman who has been on hormone therapy for a long time
- Anyone who is using or starting to use steroids

- Anyone with a condition or disease that affects bone health such as hyperthyroidism

If your bone density testing shows that you have a T-score less than –2.0, or if you have a T-score less than –1.5 and have other risk factors for osteoporosis, treatment is recommended.

Other Tests for Osteoporosis

Also available are blood and urine tests that can tell if your bones are remodeling (breaking down and building back up) at a faster-than-normal rate. Bones that remodel faster seem to be at a higher risk of fracture. However, these tests cannot tell how strong or dense your bones are and cannot be used to diagnose osteoporosis. Sometimes they are used to see if you are responding to therapy but the correlation between these tests and how your bones respond to treatment is rather weak, making this test limited in its usefulness at this time.

Treatment of Osteoporosis

If you do develop osteoporosis, calcium, vitamin D, and exercise are vital. Medications are available to help improve your bone strength. The main purpose of treatment is to prevent fractures. Besides medications, strategies to prevent falls will also help prevent fractures. Over 90 percent of hip and wrist fractures may be the result of a fall.[12]

Prevention of Falls

With age, a number of factors conspire to increase the likelihood of falling: poor vision, muscle weakness, poor balance, illnesses, and the use of certain medications. Environmental factors such as the placement of furniture can be modified to help decrease the likelihood of falls.

The following steps can be taken to help avoid falls and thus avoid fractures:

- Placing furniture to allow easy access and maneuvering
- Keeping the floors free of clutter and cords
- Placing nonslip pads under rugs

- Placing grab bars by bathtubs, showers, and toilets
- Placing night lights in bathrooms and halls
- Wearing rubber-soled, low-heeled shoes
- Avoiding walking around the house in socks
- Installing handrails on both sides of the stairs
- Placing a nonslip pad in the bathtub and shower
- Having your vision checked regularly
- Avoiding alcohol
- Exercising regularly, which improves strength and balance

Hip pads that fit under your clothing are available and provide cushioning if you do fall. This has been shown to decrease the number of hip fractures.[13] Unfortunately, they can be unattractive and uncomfortable in hot weather.

Medications for Treatment of Osteoporosis

Estrogen, bisphosphonates, selective estrogen receptor modulators, and calcitonin all help improve bone density, but they all have their advantages and disadvantages. However, they only help the bones rebuild to a certain degree. They do not make the bones return to normal.

Estrogen

Estrogen has been around for many years and has been shown to decrease bone loss and hip and spine fractures in women who have gone through menopause. Estrogen probably does this by decreasing the breakdown of bone. Estrogen has the added benefit of helping women with menopausal symptoms. However, the main downsides are an increased risk of other problems (see chapter 9).

Selective Estrogen-Receptor Modulators (SERMs)

Selective Estrogen-Receptor Modulators (SERMs) are medications that act like estrogens in one area of the body and like an antiestrogen in other parts of the body. A SERM called raloxifene (Evista) has been approved by the FDA for the prevention and treatment of osteoporosis. Raloxifene acts like an estrogen in the bone, but like an antiestrogen in the breast and uterus.

Raloxifene has also been shown to help improve bone density and reduce the likelihood of spine fractures, but not hip or other fractures in postmenopausal women.[14] It probably acts similarly to estrogen by decreasing the breakdown of bone. (See chapter 9 for more information on SERMs.)

Bisphosphonates

Bisphosphonates are a class of nonhormonal medications that bind directly to the bone to decrease its breakdown. Alendronate (Fosamax) and risedronate (Actonel) are the two that have been approved by the FDA for use in the prevention and treatment of osteoporosis. Bisphosphonates have been shown to improve bone density and decrease hip, spine, and wrist fractures. The benefit of these medications may also continue for years after they are discontinued.

Bisphosphonates do not help with menopausal symptoms. The most common complaints are stomach upset and esophagitis (inflammation in the esophagus), which can be severe in a small number of women. Because of this, women who have certain problems with their esophagus, such as esophageal strictures (where there is a narrowing of the esophagus), should avoid bisphosphonates.

Bisphosphonates are best taken in the morning on an empty stomach with eight ounces of water. You should stay upright and not eat or drink for thirty minutes after the medicine is taken. They can be taken daily or weekly, which should help with side effects.

Calcitonin

Calcitonin is a hormone that is involved in regulating calcium levels in the blood and bone metabolism. Calcitonin suppresses the breakdown of bone, thus improving bone density and reducing the risk of fractures of the spine. It also helps decrease the pain caused by fractures of the spine.

Calcitonin is taken as a nasal spray once a day. Its main side effect is irritation of the nasal passages and rarely ulceration of those passages.

The following chart compares the different medicatons used to treat osteoporosis.

Even though there are treatment options for osteoporosis, like everything else in life, an ounce of prevention is worth a pound of cure. Maintaining good bone health by taking in adequate amounts of calcium, doing daily weight-bearing exercises, and avoiding those things that are known to hurt your bones (such as smoking and alcohol) is the best way to keep your bones healthy and strong.

	Estrogen	Raloxifene	Bisphosphonates	Calcitonin
How it's given	Orally daily or by patch	Orally once a day	Orally once a day or weekly	Nasally once a day
Effect on fracture risk	Decreases hip and spine fractures	Decreases spine fractures	Decreases hip and spine fractures	Decreases spine fractures
Other benefits	Decreases menopausal symptoms	May decrease breast cancer		
Side effects	Breast tenderness, increased cardiovascular problems	Increased hot flashes, leg cramps, blood clots	Stomach upset, esophagitis	Nasal irritation
Should be avoided in people with:	Increased risk of cardiovascular problems, history of breast or uterine cancer, and increased risk of forming blood clots in their veins	Increased risk of forming blood clots in their veins	Esophageal problems	

HEART DISEASE

Heart disease and stroke are the two most common forms of cardiovascular disease. In the year 2000, cardiovascular disease killed over half a million women, while all forms of cancer combined killed 267,009 women.[15]

Heart disease is the leading killer of women in the United States and most developed countries. In 2000, heart disease claimed the lives of 254,630 women compared to 41,872 lives from breast cancer. Heart disease and stroke account for 41.3 percent of all female deaths in this country.[16] Unfortunately, there is still a misperception that heart disease is mainly a disease seen in men and not a real threat to women. This misperception isn't just among the general public but is also seen in the medical profession, potentially causing delays in this diagnosis in women.

The major risk factors for heart disease in women are cigarette smoking, high blood pressure, lipid problems, diabetes, obesity, sedentary lifestyle, and poor nutrition.[17] Other risk factors, such as a strong family history of heart disease and age (the older you are, the higher your risk of heart disease), can't be changed.

There are several warning signs of a heart attack:[18]

- Chest discomfort. Most heart attacks cause discomfort in the middle of the chest that lasts for more than a few minutes and/or can come and go. It can feel like pressure (as if someone is sitting on your chest), like your chest is being squeezed, can feel like burning, or be painful.
- Discomfort in other areas of your upper body. The discomfort or pain can go into your neck, jaw, one or both arms, back, or stomach.
- Shortness of breath. You may feel like you're having a hard time getting your breath. This may occur before or during the chest discomfort.
- Other signs. You may break out in a cold sweat or feel nauseated, lightheaded, and/or very fatigued.

The symptoms may be sudden and intense though most heart attacks start slowly and build gradually from mild symptoms. This makes it difficult to tell what's happening and can lead to delays in seeking help. Women are more likely than men to have symptoms that are not typically associated with a heart attack. Rather than chest pain, a woman may describe the sensation as a burning or fullness in the upper abdomen. This also can lead to a delay in diagnosis. If the discomfort lasts for ten to twenty minutes and is precipitated by exertion or emotional stress, it should be evaluated further by a physician.[19]

If you or someone you're with has chest discomfort, don't wait for more than a few minutes to call for help. Calling 911 is almost always the fastest way to get medical help because the emergency medical staff can start treating you right away. If you don't have access to emergency medical services, have someone else drive you to the hospital immediately.

What Causes Heart Disease?

The most common cause of heart disease is atherosclerosis, or a hardening of the arteries, which results from a buildup of plaque on the inner walls of the arteries. As the plaque builds up, the arteries become more narrow, decreasing the amount of blood that can flow through them. This decreases the amount of oxygen the artery can deliver. If this occurs in the arteries that feed the heart, you may experience some angina pectoris (chest pains) from a lack of oxygen going to the heart.

A heart attack occurs if the artery gets completely blocked, usually by a blood clot. No blood flows, cutting off the oxygen to part of the heart and that heart muscle starts to die. If only a small part of the heart is affected, you may recover and be able to improve your health, which will decrease the chance you will have another heart attack. If a larger area is damaged, you may have limitations on the activities you can perform and you may have trouble even with the activities of daily living.

What Can You Do to Decrease Your Risk of Heart Disease?

Heart disease is the number-one killer of women. Some risk factors, such as family history and age, are unalterable. If you smoke, stop. Smoking not only increases your risk for heart disease, it also increases your risk for stroke, osteoporosis, lung and other cancers, lung diseases, and other health problems. Every year, smoking kills more than 142,000 women in this country. Lung cancer now kills more women than breast cancer.[20]

The first thing you can do is calculate your risk factor for heart disease. Using the tables on pages 274–75, add up the points to see your ten-year risk for having heart disease.[21]

Your physician should address your other risk factors, such as high blood pressure, lipid problems, and diabetes. But lifestyle changes such as diet and increased activity can help significantly improve these problems. Lifestyle changes can also alter the other risk factors such as obesity, sedentary lifestyle, and poor nutrition. Even a 10 percent weight loss in obese women may significantly decrease their risk of heart disease.[22]

Let's look at three areas where you can improve your risk factor for heart disease: exercise, diet, and sleep.

Exercise

Okay, everyone knows that exercise is good for you. But what are the benefits? They include:[23]

- Strengthens the heart
- Increases muscles and strength
- Strengthens bones
- Helps control weight

- Decreases risk of diabetes
- Lowers blood pressure
- Decreases risk of colon cancer
- Improves mood, decreases anxiety and depression
- Raises HDL (the good cholesterol)
- Improves immune functioning
- Reduces the amount of fat around the waist (fat around the waist increases your risk for heart disease, diabetes, high blood pressure, and cholesterol problems)

How Much Should You Exercise?

The biggest problem with exercise is that it takes time. Your schedule is likely already overly packed. And the CDC (Centers for Disease Control and Prevention) and the American College of Sports Medicine recommend doing thirty minutes or more of moderate intensity activity on most, preferably all, days of the week.[24] When are you going to find time to exercise?

There is evidence that you don't have to do all of the activity at one time to get the benefit.[25] You can do a little here and a little there so that you get in a total of thirty minutes of daily brisk activity. That could include taking the stairs instead of the elevator or parking farther away. You could take a ten-minute walk during your lunch break. Be creative.

Of course, you don't have to stop at thirty minutes. The more active you are, the better it is for your overall health. There is a relationship between the amount of energy expended and the drop in the risk for heart disease.[26] So the more calories you burn a day, the healthier you will be. Every little bit helps.

How Hard Should You Exercise?

The other question is, How much to exert yourself in order to reap these benefits? It appears that brisk walking of at least three miles an hour (which means you will walk one mile in twenty minutes) is the minimum necessary to help decrease the risk of heart disease.[27] But before you say, "I can't do thirty minutes at this level every day" and decide to give up and do nothing, remember that some level of activity is still beneficial. More is better, but some is better than none. Make sure you don't overexert yourself from day one or you may quit before your body can get used to this new activity. Start easy and gradually build up your level of activity.

First Step:

Age (years)	Points
30–34	–9
35–39	–4
40–44	0
45–49	+3
50–54	+6
55–59	+7
60–74	+8

Second Step

Total Cholesterol (mg/dL)	Points
<160	–2
160–199	0
200–279	+1
≥280	+3

Third Step

HDL Cholesterol (mg/dL)	Points
<35	+5
35–44	+2
45–49	+1
50–59	0
≥60	–3

Fourth Step

Blood Pressure				
Systolic (mmHg) [The top number]	Diastolic (mmHg) [The bottom number]			
	<80	80–89	90–99	≥100
<120	–3	0	+2	+3
120–139	0	0	+2	+3
140–159	+2	+2	+2	+3
≥160	+3	+3	+3	+3

Fifth Step

Diabetes	Points
No	0
Yes	+4

Sixth Step

Smoker	Points
No	0
Yes	+2

Add up the points:

Age	
Total Cholesterol	
HDL Cholesterol	
Blood Pressure	
Diabetes	
Smoker	
Total Points	

Heart Disease Risk

Total Points	Your risk of having heart disease within the next ten years
≤ 2	1%
−1 to 1	2%
2 to 3	3%
4 to 5	4%
6	5%
7	6%
8	7%
9	8%
10	10%
11	11%
12	13%
13	15%
14	18%
15	20%
16	24%
≥17	≥27%

(Scoring system developed by the National Cholesterol Education Program based on the experience of the National Heart Lung and Blood Institute Framingham Heart Study.)

What Kinds of Exercise Should You Do?

Find hobbies, sports, or some activity you enjoy. If you enjoy something, you're more likely to continue to do it in the long run. It doesn't have to be expensive. Walking is one of the best things to do. It's relatively easy on the joints. It is a weight-bearing activity, which means that you carry the weight of your body, and this also helps strengthen your bones. It's free—with the exception of getting good walking shoes—and can be done anywhere.

Whether it's gardening or dancing, bowling or golf, find something you want to do and start slow. If you can only do ten minutes of walking a day, then do it. Over time, you can gradually add more activity to your life. Regular physical activity is probably the best thing you can do to help yourself stay healthier, live longer, have fewer problems, feel better, have more energy, and look better. You have to start somewhere. Start today. Start now. It's up to you.

Dietary Changes to Prevent Heart Disease

Dietary changes that may specifically help reduce your risk of heart disease include:[28]

- Substituting monounsaturated and polyunsaturated fat for saturated fat and transfatty acids (see chapter 5)
- Eating a diet high in fruits, vegetables, nuts, and whole grains (especially green leafy vegetables and foods rich in vitamin C like fruits and vegetables) and low in refined grains (such as white bread and white rice)
- Increasing fiber intake
- Increasing omega-3 fatty acids from fish or plant sources

Vitamins

Folate and vitamins B6 and E may provide some protection against heart disease and may be reasonable to take in a general multivitamin if your diet doesn't contain foods high in these vitamins. Folate is found in dark-green leafy vegetables, whole-grain cereals, and animal products. Vitamin B6 is in poultry, fish, meat, legumes, nuts, potatoes, and whole grains. And vitamin E is found in margarine, salad oils, legumes, and nuts.

Omega-3 Fatty Acids

Omega-3 fatty acids have been shown to reduce the incidence of heart disease and lower triglyceride levels. Fatty fish such as salmon, trout, and sardines tend to have higher concentrations of omega-3 fatty acids than other leaner fish.[29]

Before you decide to eat just fish all the time, bear in mind that some species of fish may contain significant levels of mercury and other environmental contaminants. The FDA recommends that pregnant or nursing women and young children should eliminate shark, swordfish, king mackerel, and tile fish from their diets completely and limit their consumption of other fish to twelve ounces per week. Other people may eat up to seven ounces of the above-mentioned fish per week.[30]

Plant sources of omega-3 fatty acids include soy foods such as tofu, walnuts, flaxseed, canola, and their oils. These foods contain alpha-linolenic acid, a type of omega-3 fatty acid. Because of the benefit for the heart, the American Heart Association now recommends that you eat at least two servings of fish (preferably fatty) a week, and that you include oils and foods rich in alpha-linolenic acid (flaxseed, canola, and soybean oils; flaxseed and walnuts).[31]

Alcohol

Wine, margaritas, beer, martinis, and other drinks are all different ways of consuming alcohol. It seems that stories pop up all the time extolling the healthful effects of alcohol, especially with respect to heart disease. Then again, you also hear about the negative effects of alcohol, such as liver problems. What should you do? Is that glass of wine with dinner okay?

As with everything else in life, the answer isn't so simple. Alcohol does seem to have some benefits: Drinking light to moderate amounts of alcohol seems to decrease the risk of heart disease and certain kinds of strokes.[32] Part of the problem is the meaning of moderate. Different studies used different levels and the beneficial amount seemed to be gender and age related. But generally, up to one alcoholic drink (one can of beer or one five-ounce glass of wine) a day seems to provide the most protection for women.[33] Higher amounts actually increase the risk of heart disease.

How the alcohol is consumed also plays a factor. When taken as part of a meal, alcohol seems to provide benefits; conversely, drinking outside of meals or drinking heavily intermittently seems to actually increase the risk of heart disease. There are some indications that wine is more protective than other types of alcohol.[34]

However, alcohol is not without problems. Alcohol also increases the risk of liver disease, certain cancers, high blood pressure, unintentional injuries, accidents, and violence.[35] Cancers of the mouth, esophagus, throat, liver, colon, and breast are higher in women who regularly drink alcohol.[36] The risk of dying from breast cancer was 30 percent higher among women reporting at least one drink a day compared to nondrinkers.[37]

Alcohol is also a source of empty calories. Each gram of alcohol has seven calories compared to four calories per gram of carbohydrates and proteins.[38] Alcohol use can also lead to excessive drinking and alcoholism. These problems entail long-term negative health and social consequences.

Compared to men, women develop alcoholic hepatitis and cirrhosis after drinking less alcohol daily and after fewer years of drinking. Drinking a glass and a half of wine or a beer and a half a day is enough to significantly increase the risk of cirrhosis in women. This amount is less than half needed to get the same negative result in men.[39]

So don't start drinking alcohol just to protect your heart or because you feel that it's good for you. Alcohol may have some benefits, but it also has a dark side. If you enjoy a glass of wine with your dinner, that's fine. Just limit your intake to no more than one glass a night. And of course if you do drink, don't drive.

Aspirin

Taking aspirin 75 mg a day has been shown to provide protection in people who are at increased risk of heart disease. This includes women who have gone through menopause and younger women with risk factors. Aspirin has also been shown to decrease the risk of colon and breast cancer as well as Alzheimer's disease.[40] However, taking aspirin (even a "baby" aspirin) increases the risk of certain strokes and bleeding from the stomach.[41] Talk to your physician to see if you should take aspirin to reduce your chances of heart disease.

Sleep

Some interesting studies have found that a lack of sleep may increase the risk of heart disease.[42] It is unclear if the lack of sleep is the cause of heart disease or that something else such as stress is causing both the lack of sleep and increase in heart disease. However, there are some intriguing studies showing that short-term sleep deprivation can raise blood pressure, lower glucose tolerance, and increase levels of stress hormones, which could explain the relationship between a lack of sleep and heart disease.[43] Until more studies are done, you should try to get an adequate amount of sleep.

STROKE

Stroke is the third leading cause of death in the United States and a leading cause of chronic disability. In 2000, 102,892 women died of stroke.[44] More women than men die of stroke.

What Causes Strokes?

A stroke occurs when the blood supply is cut off to part of the brain. When this happens, those brain cells may be permanently damaged or may die if the blood flow to that area is not restored within several minutes. The symptoms a person has with a stroke is determined by which part of the brain is affected.

There are two major types of strokes: ischemic strokes, caused by blood clots blocking the arteries feeding the brain, and hemorrhagic strokes, caused by ruptured blood vessels in the brain. The most common type of stroke is caused by blood clots that usually form in arteries damaged by atherosclerosis (a buildup of plaque in the arteries). If the blockage is temporary, it may cause a transient ischemic attack (TIA) or a "ministroke."

The risk factors for stroke include:

- Age: the older you are, the more likely you are to have a stroke
- Race: African Americans have a higher risk of stroke because of the increased incidence of high blood pressure
- Family history of stroke
- Diabetes
- High cholesterol
- High blood pressure
- Heart disease
- Being overweight
- Physical inactivity

- Smoking
- Excessive alcohol intake: drinking more than two drinks a day increases blood pressure while binge drinking can lead more directly to stroke

The warning signs of a stroke are:

- Sudden numbness or weakness of the face, arm, leg, especially if it is only on one side of the body
- Sudden confusion, trouble speaking, or understanding speech
- Sudden trouble walking, dizziness, or loss of balance or coordination
- Sudden severe headache
- Sudden trouble seeing

If you or someone you're with has any of these symptoms, don't wait for more than a few minutes to call for help. Calling 911 is almost always the fastest way to get medical help because the emergency medical staff can support you if you have problems on the way to the hospital. If you don't have access to emergency medical services, have someone else drive you to the hospital immediately.

Sometimes these symptoms may start suddenly, last for only a few minutes, and then completely resolve. This could be a TIA (transient ischemic attack), which should still be evaluated. Ten percent of people with a TIA will have a serious stroke within a year.[45]

What Can You Do to Decrease the Risk of Stroke?

Several stroke risk factors, such as age, race, and family history, cannot be changed. Of the other risk factors, high blood pressure is the biggest risk factor for stroke. This is why treatment of high blood pressure is so important. As you get older, your blood pressure gradually rises. Most people with high blood pressure feel fine. But the extra pressure on the blood vessels and heart eventually causes major problems such as stroke and heart disease.

Keeping your diabetes and cholesterol levels under good control will also help protect you against having a stroke. Lifestyle changes such as increased activity, improved diet, no smoking, and cutting back on alcohol will also help decrease your risk for stroke and improve your overall health. The dietary changes to help decrease heart disease as described earlier may also help. This is because the most common type of stroke is caused by atherosclerosis. Exercise and dietary changes may help decrease its formation. However, aspirin, which may help with heart disease and perhaps strokes caused by atherosclerosis, may actually increase the risk of hemorrhagic strokes. So discuss with your physician whether the benefits of taking aspirin outweigh its risks for you.

THE BOTTOM LINE

Health problems become more common after menopause. Some of the problems, such as osteoporosis, heart disease, and stroke, can cause significant disability, affecting your quality of life, and could lead to death. Nonetheless, getting older does not mean health problems are inevitable. There are many things you can do to keep yourself healthy and decrease the likelihood of these problems. You have a fair amount of control over your health. It's up to you to make the best of this chapter of your life.

CHAPTER 12

SCREENING TESTS

*H*ave you ever wondered exactly what your physician is doing when you see him or her? What are they looking for when they examine you and order different tests? At first, you may have been too embarrassed to ask those questions, just wanting to be done with the tests as quickly as possible. After seeing your physician for years, you felt silly asking any questions during your visits because you felt like you should know the purpose of each of the tests by now. Finally, we will lay bare the reason for each part of the exam and screening tests done when you see your physician.

THE ANNUAL EXAM

Before You See Your Physician

Once a year, you go to see your physician for your annual exam. The main part you remember is the Pap smear, which is a very important part of the visit, but only a single part of the overall visit. After the usual wait, pleasantly spent thumbing through two-year-old *Field and Stream* magazines, you will be called back. A medical assistant or nurse may get more information from you, weigh you, and obtain your blood pressure. You may be asked to leave a urine specimen and have some blood work done.

Some practices routinely test your urine for the presence of certain things such as blood, white blood cells, sugar, and other things. Other practices do not routinely test the urine because there is no strong evidence that screening women who are not having any urinary problems is effective at picking up any major problems.

Ask Questions

When you see your physician, he or she may ask you questions. This is the best time to voice any concerns you may have. If you don't speak up, your physician may have no idea that something may be worrying you, whether it is about a possible lump you may have felt in your breast, anxiety symptoms, fatigue, leakage of urine, or a drop in your libido. Write down your questions before your visit so you don't forget what to ask. Many women feel uncomfortable talking about certain issues, but this is probably one of the best places to get advice on those issues that are bothering you.

The Exam

Next comes the examination. Different physicians do this differently. You may find this surprising, but there is no "standard" way of doing a physical exam. Even the different parts of the exam, such as the breast or pelvic exams, may be done differently by different physicians.

Head and Neck

Starting from the top, you may have your eyes, ears, mouth, and throat examined. The lymph nodes in your neck and the area above the collarbone (also called the clavicle) may be felt to see if they are abnormally enlarged, which may be a sign of infection or rarely of some type of cancer.

The thyroid is in the front part of your neck and may be felt to see if it is enlarged or if there are any nodules. An enlarged thyroid is called a goiter and may be a sign that your thyroid is under- or overactive. A nodule on the thyroid may be a benign cyst or may be a cancer.

The Breast Exam

The breast exam may be done while you are sitting and/or lying on your back. One breast may be slightly larger than the other. Your physician will note any skin changes or dimpling. Any unusual lumps will be evaluated further. If you have noted any changes in your breasts or nipple discharge, this is the time to bring it to your physician's attention. This way, you can pinpoint the lump or abnormality you feel and make sure that your physician is feeling what you are feeling. After all, you know your body better than anyone else.

The Pelvic Exam

Your abdomen may be palpated to see if there are any unusual growths. During the pelvic exam, the outer part of the genital area called the vulva is examined to see if there are any unusual growths or moles. Your physician may have you bear down to see if your bladder or rectum bulges significantly toward the vaginal opening.

The speculum (hopefully after it has been warmed) is placed into the vagina to be able to see the cervix. The speculum is a metal or plastic instrument shaped like a long narrow duckbill that opens up to separate the vaginal walls so that the vagina and cervix can be seen. The cervix is at the top of the vagina and is the bottom part of the uterus. It looks like a small pink doughnut with a very small hole. The vaginal walls and cervix are also examined for any unusual features.

The Pap smear is done by collecting cervical cells with a spatula and a brush. This may cause some cramping and spotting, especially when the brush is placed in your cervical canal to collect the endocervical cells (cells that line the cervical canal).

After the Pap smear is completed, your physician will place one or two fingers inside your vagina and the other hand on your abdomen in order to feel your uterus and ovaries. He or she can tell whether your uterus is tipped forward or backward, the size of the uterus, and if it contains any sizable fibroids.

Most women have a uterus that is tipped forward where it sits on the bladder. Some women have a uterus that is tipped backward; in other words, the top of the uterus is leaning toward the back. A uterus that is tipped backward usually doesn't cause any problems except that it may make deep penetration with intercourse more uncomfortable in some women. It used to be thought that a uterus tipped backward made it harder to get pregnant, though this is not true.

An enlarged uterus may be a sign of fibroids (benign growths on the uterus) or adenomyosis, which is a condition in which part of the lining of the uterus (the endometrium) grows into the uterine walls. Rarely, an enlarged uterus could be a sign of a cancer growing in the uterus. (See chapter 3 for more information on these conditions.)

Any major growths on your ovaries may also be detected by this exam. This could represent a simple cyst, which your ovaries produce every month when you ovulate. These cysts may be detected on a pelvic exam and can be confirmed by ultrasound. Benign tumors or cancers can also cause a growth on the ovary.

A number of factors such as a thicker waistline or tensing the stomach muscles may affect the ability of your physician to pick up any changes on your ovaries or uterus. Other areas of the pelvis may also be evaluated such as the area behind the uterus and different glands in the vagina. Your physician may also test the strength of your pelvic floor by having you do your Kegel's exercise (tightening the muscles around the opening of your vagina).

Rectal Exam

A rectal exam may or may not be done. Some providers do them on everyone. Others only do them once you reach a certain age such as forty or fifty because that's when there is a rise in incidence of colorectal cancer. Its purpose is to detect any abnormal growths in the rectum such as a polyp or cancer and to test for blood in the stool. Blood in the stool may indicate a problem such as colon polyps, cancer, or ulcers.

After the exam, your physician may order other tests such as a mammogram, a bone density test, and blood tests for cholesterol and diabetes. (Some of these tests will be described in more detail below.)

CERVICAL CANCER SCREENING

An estimated 12,900 new cases of cervical cancer were diagnosed in the United States in 2001.[1] Fortunately, this number has been significantly lowered by the advent of the Pap smear. (See chapter 8 under human papillomavirus for more information about cervical cancer screening.)

ENDOMETRIAL (UTERINE) CANCER SCREENING

Endometrial cancer is the most common gynecologic cancer in this country, with an estimated 38,300 new cases in 2001. Fortunately, most of these women will be cured and only 6,600 deaths will be caused by this cancer.[2] The reason for the high cure rate is that most endometrial cancers are caught early. Endometrial cancer has early symptoms, mainly abnormal bleeding from the uterus, which prompts an evaluation. When the cancer is discovered, it is usually still confined to the uterus and has not spread, which leads to the high cure rates. (See chapter 3 for more information about endometrial cancer.)

OVARIAN CANCER SCREENING

Ovarian cancer kills more women in this country than all other gynecologic cancers combined, with approximately 23,400 new cases of ovarian cancer in 2001 and 13,900 deaths.[3] Unfortunately, 70 percent of women with ovarian cancer are diagnosed when their disease is already at an advanced stage, leading to a poor 28 percent five-year survival rate. If the ovarian cancer is caught early and is confined to the ovaries, the survival rate is around 95 percent.[4]

Ovarian cancers are not caught early for a number of reasons. First, the ovaries are relatively inaccessible and are difficult to examine directly. Additionally, most ovarian cancers do not cause any symptoms such as pain when they are small. If they do cause symptoms, they are usually vague and not specific. By the time they do cause significant symptoms, they have already grown and spread.

Risk Factors for Ovarian Cancer

Most women with ovarian cancer have no identifiable risk factor. However, up to 10 percent of the most common type of ovarian cancer, called epithelial ovarian cancer, is related to an inherited gene mutation.[5] The most common mutation is seen in the BRCA1 and BRCA2 genes. In those women with a BRCA1 mutation, they have a 16 to 40 percent chance of developing ovarian cancer in their lifetime.[6] Because of this high risk, many women with the BRCA1 mutation choose to have their ovaries removed once they have finished having children to reduce their chances of getting ovarian cancer. But as described later, this does not eliminate the risk. Genetic testing can be done to see if you have this mutation (see below).

Other minor risk factors include a personal history of breast, colon, or endometrial cancer; bearing no children; and living in North America or northern Europe.[7] The use of any birth control pills decreases the risk of ovarian cancer.[8]

CA-125 and Pelvic Ultrasound

The tests currently used to detect ovarian cancer, CA-125 and pelvic ultrasound, are limited. CA-125 is a blood test that can detect ovarian cancer. The main problems with the test are its low sensitivity and specificity. In other words, the CA-125 misses up to half of early ovarian cancers.[9] It is also less likely to detect a smaller ovarian cancer at an early stage. The other problem is that a number of benign conditions such as endometriosis and fibroids can raise the CA-125 levels.[10] CA-125 can also detect peritoneal cancers (cancer of the lining of the pelvis and abdomen described below under genetic testing). So, the CA-125 test is not a good screening test because it can be elevated with other benign conditions and it isn't significantly elevated in many cases until ovarian cancer has already spread.

Using a pelvic ultrasound to look at the ovaries has also been studied as a screening tool for ovarian cancer. Ultrasound seems to be able to detect ovarian cancers earlier, but it also picks up a number of benign changes in the ovaries. The biggest problem with a positive CA-125 or pelvic ultrasound is that the only way to determine if there really is ovarian cancer is to do surgery. That is the other cost of screening. Of the women with a pelvic ultrasound suspicious for ovarian cancer, ten to eleven would have to undergo surgery in order to find one cancer.[11] In other words, when the ultrasound picks up something suspicious, it is an ovarian cancer only about 10 percent of the time, thus subjecting 90 percent of these women to unnecessary surgery with its risks.

So currently, there are no good screening tests for ovarian cancer for the general population. Other promising tests are being developed that may become available in the future. For those women at high risk for ovarian cancer, a combination of pelvic ultrasound and CA-125 may be used, though their use is of limited value.

BREAST CANCER SCREENING

Breast cancer is the second leading cause of death from cancer in women in the United States (second only to lung cancer). One out of thirty women will die of breast cancer.[12] Breast cancer screening is best done by using three approaches: (1) monthly self-breast exams (right after your period if you are still having them because that's when the lumpiness in your breast is least prominent), (2) yearly clinical breast exams done by your physician, and (3) mammograms.

Mammograms

Mammograms should be done every one to two years from ages forty to fifty and yearly after fifty. Since not all breast cancers can be detected by mammogram, suspicious masses felt on exam should evaluated further even if the mammogram is normal.

Mammography uses X-rays to penetrate the breast as it is flattened between two plates. The X-rays have a harder time passing through a growth in the breast, which causes a shadow that can be seen on the X-ray picture. Flattening the breasts allows the X-rays to penetrate the breast tissue more easily and makes it more easy to detect masses in the breast. The more the breast is flattened the better the X-ray pictures, but unfortunately, the more uncomfortable it is. A mammogram can detect not only masses in the breast by their shadows, but also some breast cancers that have distinct-looking calcium deposits.

Recently, some studies have thrown doubt on the effectiveness of mammogram and self-breast exam to detect breast cancer early enough to make a difference. However, the majority of studies show mammography as an effective tool to detect breast cancer. Though mammogram is far from a perfect test, missing up to 30 percent of breast cancers, it is still the only screening test available for breast cancer.[13]

The main downside is that mammograms can also see suspicious areas that turn out to be benign changes. Unfortunately, if you have a suspicious finding, you may go through a period of worry as well as the pain and risks of a biopsy only to find out that there was nothing bad there in the first place. Mammograms can also give you a false sense of security. A normal mammogram is reassuring, but since mammograms can miss a cancer, any suspicious or new lump you feel should be evaluated.

Other Breast Tests

Other tests such as MRI (magnetic resonance imaging) and thermal scanning are still experimental. Ultrasound is used as a diagnostic tool to evaluate masses felt on an exam or seen on a mammogram to determine if it is solid or filled with fluid. This can help with diagnosis, but has not been shown to be effective as a screening test in women without symptoms. Mammogram is also less effective in younger women. This is because women who have not gone through menopause—especially those under forty—tend to have denser breasts, making it harder for the mammogram to pick up any abnormalities.

Self-Breast Exams

Self-breast exams have also been questioned for their effectiveness. For years, many physicians and organizations have recommended women routinely examine their breasts. It may come as a surprise that its effectiveness is still unclear. Currently, there is insufficient evidence to encourage or discourage women from doing self-breast exams.

However, you may be able to detect a new lump between your annual visits and mammograms, and since it is not painful, is free, and is easy to do, self-breast exams are a reasonable practice to continue. Self-breast exams are not perfect. No screening test is. You may still miss a new lump, but if you don't examine your breasts, then you won't pick up anything until it becomes obvious.

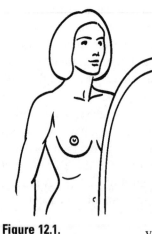

Doing your breast exam is sometimes a confusing task. You think you are supposed to find lumps in your breast, but your breasts always feel lumpy. That's the way they're supposed to feel. Your breasts are made of two parts, the fatty part that makes your breasts soft and the deeper glandular tissue that produces milk. The glandular part is what feels lumpy and changes with your cycles because of the hormonal changes.

The best time to do your breast exam is right after your period has ended. That's when your breasts are the least lumpy. Before your period, the rising hormone levels tend to

Figure 12.1.

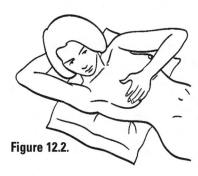

Figure 12.2.

make your breasts more tender and lumpy.

Do your breast exam before and during bathing. That way, you are already undressed. Look at your breasts in the mirror. One breast may be slightly larger than the other, which is normal. Look for any dimpling or puckering of the skin, changes in size or shape of the breast, or nipple discharge.

You may want to lie down and place one arm behind your head. If you can, place a pillow under that shoulder. All of these things help flatten your breast tissue over your chest wall, making it easier to feel if something new is present.

Use the part of your three middle fingers where your fingerprints are to do the exam. Feel your breast tissue using circular motions about the size of a dime and varying the amount of pressure: first use light pressure to feel near the surface, then medium to feel in between, and deep pressure to feel deep into the breast. You can examine your breasts in a circular pattern, going from the outside and working your way to the nipple or up and down in lines. Whichever

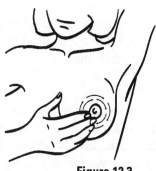

Figure 12.3.

way you use, just make sure to examine the whole breast all the way to the armpit and collarbone.

You can also examine your breasts in the shower. The soapy water sometimes makes it easier to feel anything unusual.

You are not feeling for lumps in your breasts, since your breasts are naturally lumpy. What you are really feeling for are changes in your breasts. If you examine your breasts regularly, you will get to know what is normal for you and if there is a change, that is what you bring to the attention of your physician.

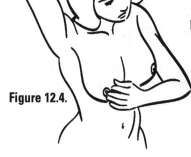

Figure 12.4.

COLON CANCER SCREENING

Colorectal cancer (cancer of the colon and rectum) is the third most common cancer in women and is the third most common cause of death, killing about twenty-nine thousand women a year.[14]

The risk factors of colorectal cancer:

- First degree relative (sibling or parent) with colorectal cancer or polyp
- Familial colorectal cancer syndromes
- Being older than fifty years of age
- History of inflammatory bowel disease (ulcerative colitis or Crohn's disease)
- History of colon polyps or colorectal cancer
- History of endometrial, breast, or ovarian cancer
- Diet high in fat or low in fiber
- Smoking
- Obesity

Unfortunately, you can't change most of these risk factors. However, the risk factors you can change are good to do so for other reasons. Increasing the fiber in your diet, cutting back on fat, stopping smoking, and bringing your weight closer to your ideal body weight will help decrease your risk for colorectal cancer as well as other life-threatening diseases. Taking aspirin regularly has been shown to decrease the risk of colon cancer.[15] Because aspirin may have certain risks, you should talk to your physician first to see if you should take it.

The likelihood of having colorectal cancers increases with age and occurs mostly over the age of fifty. For this reason, screening for colorectal cancer is recommended for all women starting at age fifty. For women with higher risk such as having a parent or sibling with colorectal cancer or polyps, the screening may be started at an earlier age. Screening helps to detect colorectal cancers earlier. Most of these cancers arise from polyps and can slowly progress to cancer. Removing the polyps prevents the cancer from developing in the first place. Screening can also pick up cancers at an earlier stage, which leads to higher cure rates.

What Are the Screening Tests Recommended to Detect Colon Cancer?

According to the American Cancer Society, beginning at age fifty, one of five screening options should be selected:[16]

- Yearly fecal occult blood testing
- Flexible sigmoidoscopy every five years
- Combination of yearly fecal occult blood testing and flexible sigmoidoscopy every five years
- Colonoscopy every ten years
- Double-contrast barium enema every five years

A digital rectal examination should be performed at the time of each screening by sigmoidoscopy, colonoscopy, or double-contrast barium enema. Advantages and disadvantages exist for each of the screening options. For example, fecal occult blood testing is the least risky, but misses the most cancers. Which screening regimen you choose depends on your risk factors, access to specialists who can perform the screening tests, and your own personal preferences.

Fecal Occult Blood Test

Three cards are given to you on which you smear a small sample of stool from three different bowel movements. You send the cards back to your physician, who tests it for tiny amounts of blood. If blood is found, you should see a gastroenterologist (a physician who specializes in the digestive tract) for further testing to find the source of the blood.

This test is not that sensitive, picking up about half of colon cancers.[17] And a number of things not related to cancers or polyps can make the test turn positive, so a positive result does not necessarily mean that you have something as serious as cancer. It just means that you need to have it evaluated to see where the blood is coming from. Though this test may miss a number of cancers, it may be useful in areas where access to the other screening tests is limited.

Sigmoidoscopy

Sigmoidoscopy is a procedure done usually at your doctor's office. The sigmoidoscope is a long, flexible tube with a light on the end. Your doctor can look through the sigmoidoscope and see your rectum and lower colon. The sigmoidoscope is placed in the rectum and advanced up your colon. The rectum and lower third of your colon can be examined this way. Sigmoidoscopy identifies 70 to 80 percent of polyps or cancers.[18]

Before going for this test, you need to clean out your colon completely so that the colon walls can be clearly seen. Different ways of cleaning out your colon are available but you need to follow the directions and do everything as directed. If not, some stool may be left in your colon and block the view. A polyp or cancer could then be missed.

Risks of Sigmoidoscopy

A sigmoidoscopy is somewhat uncomfortable, causing some cramping. Usually, no anesthesia or pain medications are given for this procedure. In one study, 14 percent reported moderate pain and 0.4 percent severe pain. A quarter of patients had gas or flatus, while 3 percent had bleeding.[19] The most serious complication of a sigmoidoscopy is perforation of the bowel, where a hole is made in the bowel. However, this is very rare, occuring in about one to two (or even less) per ten thousand procedures.[20] For any surgery or procedure, it is best to select a physician who has performed the procedure many times.

Colonoscopy

Colonoscopy is similar to sigmoidoscopy, but uses a longer tube in order to see your entire colon. This is the main advantage of colonoscopy over sigmoidoscopy, because some colon polyps and cancers can grow further up the colon beyond the view of the sigmoidoscope. Colonoscopy picks up 90 percent of polyps larger than a centimeter and about 75 percent of polyps smaller than a centimeter.[21]

You will need to clean out your colon completely before this test as for sigmoidoscopy. Make sure you follow all the directions to make sure all the stool is cleared out. Otherwise, the remaining stool may cover a polyp or cancer and it may be missed.

Colonoscopy is done in a doctor's procedure room or in the operating room. Because colonoscopy is more uncomfortable than sigmoidoscopy, it is usually done with some sedation given through an intravenous line. You will be monitored during the procedure. Because of the medications given, you will need someone to drive you home after the procedure.

Risks of Colonoscopy

The risks are higher with colonoscopy because it is a more invasive procedure and because of the sedation used. Part of the increased risk is due to the use of colonoscopy to not only look inside the colon, but to also remove polyps that are found. The risk of perforating the bowel is higher when polyps are removed or a biopsy is taken. There are about two to three major complications out of one thousand screening colonoscopies; the most common is bleeding, which may require hospitalization or emergency care.[22]

Advantages of Colonoscopy

The advantage of colonoscopy, however, is that everything can be done at once. If any of the other screening tests find something like a polyp, you would have to undergo a colonoscopy. When you have a colonoscopy as your screening test, if something is found, it can usually be removed and dealt with at the same time, potentially saving you from undergoing two procedures. The other advantage is that a colonoscopy can evaluate the entire colon.

Double-Contrast Barium Enema

Double-contrast barium enema is an X-ray test that looks at the colon in order to find polyps, diverticulosis (outpouchings from the colon wall), and other abnormalities. It is performed in the radiology department. Before the procedure, you have to clean out your colon completely. Again, if any stool is left behind, it can either hide something or make the radiologist think that there is something in your colon when it is really a piece of stool.

A tube is placed in your rectum and a balloon on the tip is inflated to hold it in place. A thick white substance containing barium is placed through the tube into your rectum. The barium is what shows up on the X-ray pictures. You will be asked to move from side to side to help the barium completely coat your colon. The radiologist will be watching on a monitor. Once the colon is filled with the barium, he or she will let most of it drain out, leaving a film of barium covering the colon walls. Air is then pumped through the tube into the colon, inflating it like a long narrow balloon.

On the monitor, the radiologist sees the outline of the colon walls and can look for any polyps, outpouchings, or other abnormalities of the colon walls. You will be asked to move into different positions to get a clearer view of different parts of the colon. Several X-ray pictures will be taken of different areas to review after the procedure. You will be asked to hold your breath while the pictures are taken to prevent the picture from becoming blurry from the movement of breathing.

Downsides of Double-Contrast Barium Enema

You may feel cramping and the urge to have a bowel movement during the procedure. After the procedure, you may feel bloated and crampy for the rest of the day. You will notice your stools looking white as your body gets rid of the barium after the procedure.

Major complications of any type occurred in one of ten thousand barium enema procedures. Perforation of the bowel is rare, occurring in one out of twenty-five thousand procedures.[23]

One study compared the accuracy of this test to colonoscopy and showed that double-contrast barium enema picked up only 24 to 67 percent of polyps seen on colonoscopy.[24] Concern that double-contrast barium enema missed a significant number of even the larger polyps may limit the usefulness of this test as a screening tool. However, it may be a useful option in vicinities where access to sigmoidoscopy and colonoscopy is limited.

CHOLESTEROL SCREENING

Heart disease is the number-one cause of death in women in this country. Cholesterol has been linked to atherosclerosis (hardening of the arteries), heart disease, stroke, and Alzheimer's disease. More and more attention is being focused on controlling cholesterol in order to decrease the risk of heart disease. According to the National Center for Health Statistics data from 1988 to 1994, 20 percent of women from ages twenty to seventy-four had high cholesterol levels (240 mg/dl or higher).[25]

Different guidelines exist as to the frequency of cholesterol testing but the National Heart, Lung, and Blood Institute recommends that testing should be done every five years starting at age twenty.[26] Ideally, a fasting lipid panel, which is a battery of blood tests for total cholesterol, LDL cholesterol (the "bad" cholesterol), HDL cholesterol (the "good" cholesterol), and triglycerides (another kind of fat in the blood), would be performed. The blood is drawn after nine to twelve hours of fasting (no eating or drinking anything except water).

If you have any of the following risk factors, you should definitely have your lipid panel tested because you are at higher risk for having high cholesterol and developing heart disease:

- Smoker
- High blood pressure (even if it is well controlled with medications)
- Diabetes
- Family history of early heart disease (heart disease in father or brother before age fifty-five or mother or sister before age sixty-five)
- Parent or sibling with elevated cholesterol

Treatment of High Cholesterol

Diet and Weight Loss

Treatment of high cholesterol for five to seven years decreases the risk of heart disease by 30 percent.[27] Changes in diet are the first line of treatment. A healthy diet, high in fruits and vegetables and low in saturated fat, as well as regular physical activity is recommended. Reducing the amount of saturated fats as well as weight loss can lower the total cholesterol and LDL by as much as 10 to 20 percent. However, most people are only able to achieve a 2 to 6 percent drop in their cholesterol levels by modifying their lifestyles.[28]

If you are unable to maintain or reduce your cholesterol level sufficiently through dietary changes, weight loss, and regular activity, medications may be necessary. A number of cholesterol-lowering medications are available and are very effective, but may have side effects.

Niacin

Niacin (nicotinic acid) is a B vitamin that can decrease your total cholesterol, LDL, and triglyceride levels while raising your HDL level. Large doses need to be taken and should be done *only* under the supervision of your physician because of potential risks. The most common side effects are hot flashes or flushing, nausea, vomiting, diarrhea, indigestion, and gas.

More serious side effects include activation of stomach ulcers, liver problems, gout, and high blood sugar.

Statins

This class of drugs slows down the production of cholesterol and increases the clearing of LDL cholesterol from the blood. Statins such as lovastatin (Mevacor), pravastatin (Pravachol), simvastatin (Zocor), fluvastatin (Lescol), atorvastatin (Lipitor), and cerivastatin (Baycol) can lower the LDL cholesterol by 20 to 60 percent and have been shown to decrease the number of heart attacks.[29] They also decrease the triglyceride levels. Most people tolerate statins well with few having upset stomach, constipation, and gas. Rarely, statins can cause liver and muscle problems that can be serious. Statins have become the most commonly used medication to treat high cholesterol because of their effectiveness and few side effects.

Bile Acid Sequestrants

Bile acid sequestrants such as cholestyramine (Questran), colestipol (Colestid), and colesevelam (WelChol) bind to cholesterol-containing bile acids in the intestines. Since they are not absorbed by the intestines, they drag the cholesterol in bile acids out of the body. This decreases LDL by 10 to 20 percent.[30] They are sometimes combined with statins to drop the cholesterol even further. The main side effects are constipation, bloating, nausea, and gas.

You will need to follow up with your physician to determine which treatment is best for you among all of these options.

DIABETES SCREENING

Diabetes is an unfortunate consequence of the developed world. As living standards improve, there is a decrease in activity levels and an increase in obesity, leading to the increase in diabetes. In 1897, diabetes was considered a rare disease, affecting only 2.8 out of 100,000 people in this country. In 1995, diabetes affected over 7 percent (or 7,000 out of 100,000 people) of adults in the United States and continues to rise. Sixteen million Americans have diabetes, but only half have been diagnosed. Another 22 million have impaired glucose tolerance (a condition where the body has higher than normal sugar levels but does not quite meet the definition of diabetes), and will probably become diabetic if untreated.[31]

What Is Diabetes?

What is diabetes? Diabetes is a disease that leads to high sugar levels, either because the body does not make enough insulin, the insulin that is made does not work well, or a combination of both. There are two types of diabetes: type 1 usually shows up in children and younger adults, and type 2 is found mostly in older adults. Type 1 diabetes is more serious and is caused by the pancreas producing inadequate amounts of insulin. Over 90 percent of diabetes in this country is type 2 diabetes and this is the type we will focus on.[32]

Risks of Diabetes

Diabetes is the seventh leading cause of death in the United States, contributing to roughly 160,000 deaths each year.[33] Diabetes increases the risk of heart attack and stroke, and is the leading cause of kidney failure and blindness in this country. However, type 2 diabetes often has no symptoms in its early stages and may be missed for many years. The problem with diabetes is the fact that high sugar levels can lead to damage of the kidneys, eyes, nerves, heart, and blood vessels. The damage diabetes causes to the nerves and blood vessels leads to injuries and infections of the feet and legs, which sometimes have to be amputated.

Screening for Diabetes

Despite all these serious consequences, as many as eight million people do not know they have diabetes. Treatment of the diabetes with good control of the sugar levels significantly decreases the likelihood of these serious problems from occurring. So who should be screened?

Unfortunately, screening everyone does not seem to be cost effective according to existing studies. The American Diabetes Association recommends that screening should be considered for individuals starting at age forty-five because the risk of diabetes increases significantly after that age and should be done every three years.

Testing should be done at a younger age or more frequently if individuals have one or more of the following risk factors:[34]

- Family history of diabetes (i.e., parents or siblings with diabetes)
- Overweight (body mass index or BMI greater than or equal to 25 kg/m^2; see chapter 5 for more information)
- Habitual physical inactivity
- Race/ethnicity (e.g., African Americans, Hispanic Americans, Native Americans, Asian Americans, and Pacific Islanders)
- Previously identified as having impaired fasting glucose or impaired glucose tolerance
- High blood pressure
- HDL cholesterol less than or equal to 35 mg/dl and/or a triglyceride level greater than or equal to 250 mg/dl
- History of gestational diabetes (diabetes during pregnancy) or delivery of a baby weighing more than nine pounds
- Polycystic ovary syndrome

The most common way to screen for diabetes is to check a fasting glucose level. You cannot eat or drink anything except for water for eight hours before the test. Your blood is drawn and sent to the lab. A fasting plasma glucose level of less than 110 mg/dl is considered normal; over 125 mg/dl is considered to be diabetes and a value between the two is considered impaired fasting glucose or impaired glucose tolerance.[35]

If there is a question about the results, or if diabetes is still suspected despite the result of the fasting glucose test, a more involved test may be done. After your fasting glucose level is drawn, you are given a very sweet drink containing seventy-five grams of glucose. Your blood is drawn two hours later and if this plasma glucose level is 200 mg/dl or higher, it means you have diabetes.[36]

OSTEOPOROSIS SCREENING

Osteoporosis is a disease of the bones that causes them to become so thin and brittle that they break very easily. Even minor stress such as coughing or sitting too hard can lead to a fracture. The bones become thinner with age and the bone loss increases after menopause. Osteoporosis is mainly seen in postmenopausal women. (For more information on osteoporosis and the different screening tests, see chapter 11.)

GENETIC TESTING

A number of cancers tend to run in families and researchers are now focusing in on changes in certain genes that may cause an increased risk of various cancers. Even though people who carry certain genetic mutations are at higher risk of certain cancers, most cancers are not caused by these specific genetic mutations. The main way of identifying if you are at increased risk for cancer is through family history.

However, the accuracy of family history is diminished beyond first-degree relatives (parents, siblings, and children). Also, gynecologic cancers are commonly mistaken for each other. For example, a woman may think her mother's grandmother had a hysterectomy for one type of gynecologic cancer such as endometrial cancer when in fact she had cervical cancer or cervical dysplasia or perhaps no cancer at all. Not uncommonly, people may misinterpret the reason for their surgery. They may hear words such as "an abnormal growth" as the reason for surgery and think it means they have a cancer when in fact they have a benign growth such as a fibroid. The best way to determine your family history is to get medical records, surgical notes, pathology reports, and death certificates to establish an accurate family history.

Hereditary Breast and Ovarian Cancer

In the mid-1990s, the BRCA1 and BRCA2 genes were identified. These genes, when normal, appear to suppress tumors. A mutation in these genes increases the risk of breast and ovarian cancers and can be passed on to the children. Some families have mostly breast cancers, while others have mostly ovarian cancers, and still others have a combination of both cancers. About 5 to 10 percent of ovarian and breast cancers are related to one of these inherited cancer syndromes.[37]

Risk of Cancer with BRCA1 and BRCA2 Mutations

People with BRCA1 and BRCA2 mutations also have a higher risk for prostate cancer (something women don't have to worry about), Fallopian tube, and primary peritoneal cancer (cancer of the lining of the pelvis and abdomen). Families with BRCA2 mutations also have an increased risk for pancreatic cancer, melanoma (a skin cancer), stomach cancer, and cholangiocarcinoma (cancer of the bile duct).

Just because you have the mutation does not mean you will have cancer. For carriers of the BRCA1 and BRCA2 mutations there is an estimated 40 to 85 percent lifetime chance of breast cancer. BRCA1 carriers have a 16 to 40 percent lifetime risk of ovarian cancer, which is higher than the 10 to 20 percent risk seen in BRCA2 carriers. BRCA1 carriers also have their ovarian cancer show up eight to fourteen years earlier than BRCA2 carriers.[38]

Testing for BRCA1 and BRCA2 Mutations

Genetic testing for BRCA1 and BRCA2 mutations is available but expensive, costing about $2,500. The test may or may not be covered by insurance. Unfortunately, the genetic testing misses about 15 percent of the mutations.[39] So a negative result does not completely let you off the hook. The test may also be indeterminate, which may cause a great deal of distress.

Who would be a good candidate for BRCA1 and BRCA 2 testing is still unclear. Women with strong family histories of breast, ovarian, colon, pancreatic, and prostate cancers; Ashkenazi Jews; and women who have had breast cancer before age forty and/or ovarian cancer before age fifty are at higher risk of carrying mutations on these genes and would be potential candidates for genetic testing.

What If You Are a Carrier?

Since being a carrier of the mutation does not necessarily mean that you will get these cancers, the question becomes, What do you do if you are a carrier? For ovarian cancer, you may opt to be screened. But screening for ovarian cancer is still quite poor.

Some women choose to have both ovaries removed to decrease the risk of ovarian cancer. However, this causes women to go through surgical menopause, which is generally more intense than natural menopause. The removal of the ovaries also is not a 100 percent guarantee that you will not get ovarian cancer and does have the risks of surgery. (See chapter 3 for more information about the risks and benefits of removing your ovaries.)

Because of this, some experts recommend checking a CA-125 test even though it is not very good at detecting these cancers. Birth control pills have been shown to decrease the risk of ovarian cancer by about 50 percent and would be reasonable to use in healthy women who need contraception.[40] Recent studies show no increase in risk of breast cancer in women taking oral contraceptives.[41]

Tamoxifen, an antiestrogen, has been shown to decrease the risk of breast cancers in high risk women by almost 50 percent.[42] This reduction was seen only in breast cancers that had estrogen receptors. Estrogen may bind to these estrogen receptors, which are on the surface of the breast cancer cells, and stimulate those cells that have these receptors to grow. Tamoxifen acts like an antiestrogen and may help block the effect of estrogen on these breast cancer cells and help the body destroy these cells.

It is unclear if this protective effect would apply to women with BRCA1 and BRCA2 mutations. Most BRCA1-related breast cancers do not have estrogen receptors and may not be responsive to tamoxifen. Currently, there are no recommendations regarding the use of tamoxifen to help prevent breast cancers in carriers of these mutations.

Removal of the ovaries before menopause has been shown to decrease the risk of breast cancers by up to 50 percent.[43] This causes menopause with its own set of issues. Some women even choose to have both breasts removed. Though drastic, prophylactic mastectomy reduces the risk of breast cancer by at least 90 percent.[44] It is still not a 100 percent guarantee and does have surgical risks as well as possible psychological consequences. On the other hand, breast cancer screening and close monitoring may not catch the breast cancer early enough to prevent death and there is the emotional burden of living with this uncertainty.[45]

Hereditary Nonpolyposis Colorectal Cancer

Hereditary nonpolyposis colorectal cancer (HNPCC) is related to a mutation in a set of genes and causes an increased risk of cancers in the colon, uterus, ovary, stomach, ureter (the tube that connects the kidney to the bladder), kidney, small intestine, brain, and bile ducts. Genetic testing probably identifies the mutation in 50 to 60 percent of families with HNPCC.[46]

Risk of Cancer

Carriers of this mutation have about an 80 percent lifetime risk of getting colorectal cancer. Colonoscopy to screen for this is recommended every one to two years beginning at age twenty-five. Endometrial cancer (cancer of the lining of the uterus) is the second most common cancer in families with HNPCC after colorectal cancer, with a lifetime risk of 40 to 60 percent. Endometrial biopsy should be done yearly beginning at age thirty. Ovarian cancer may occur in 9 percent of carriers of this mutation.[47]

Because of the increased risks of endometrial and ovarian cancers, some women choose to have their uterus and ovaries removed after they have finished having children.

It is unclear whether breast cancer is increased in these families. At a minimum, women should begin annual mammography starting at age forty. Other possible screening tests would include endoscopy (similar to a colonoscopy except the lighted tube goes through your mouth, down your throat to look inside your stomach) to screen for stomach cancer, kidney ultrasound and urine testing for kidney and ureteral cancers, and ultrasound of the gallbladder and bile ducts to screen for cancers in that area.[48]

Because of the lack of information about the effectiveness of screening and treatment strategies for women with BRCA1, BRCA2, and other mutations, some experts recommend that genetic testing be done in a research setting so that long-term data could be obtained and analyzed.[49] It is also still unclear why some people who have these genetic mutations have no cancer while others do, and what kinds of changes these people can make to reduce their risk of cancer.

Should You Have Genetic Testing?

Whether or not you should have genetic testing is another question. Potentially, a positive result could affect your ability to obtain health, life, and disability insurance and may have an effect on your employment. It may also cause anxiety or depression. Moreover, a positive result does not mean that you will definitely have a cancer in the future; it just increases that chance.

However, if you do have a positive result, you may choose to take medications or have surgery to decrease your risk and/or have certain screening tests done. You should consider talking to a genetic counselor and carefully weigh the risks and benefits before you choose to have testing performed.

SCREENING FOR THYROID DISEASE

The thyroid gland is located on the front of the lower part of your neck. Thyroid means oblong shield and was named by Thomas Wharton in 1656.[50] The thyroid gland produces thyroid hormones that regulate your body's metabolism.

The thyroid gland can cause problems by either producing too much thyroid hormones, called hyperthyroidism, or not enough, which is hypothyroidism. Both hyperthyroidism and hypothyroidism are more common in women than men and more common as you get older.

Hypothyroidism

Women with hypothyroidism can feel sluggish, tired, and depressed because they have low thyroid levels. Their metabolism slows, causing a number of symptoms that can be confused with symptoms of aging. Women can have irregular periods or no periods at all (see chapter 3). They can also have problems with:

- fatigue
- weight gain
- dry skin
- constipation
- cold intolerance (cold bothers them more now than in the past)
- poor concentration and memory

Hypothyroidism can also be confused with depression. If you have any of these symptoms, you should be tested. Hypothyroidism can be detected by testing your blood for thyroid stimulating hormone (TSH). TSH is the hormone that stimulates your thyroid to produce thyroid hormones. If your thyroid is not making enough thyroid hormones, the TSH goes up, trying to get the thyroid to produce more. So an elevated TSH means that your thyroid levels are low and you have hypothyroidism.

Hypothyroidism can not only make you feel fatigued, it can also cause high blood pressure, increased cholesterol, anemia, and affect your heart. Treatment is straightforward. You simply take thyroid hormones in a pill and adjust the dose until your TSH is in the normal range.

Hyperthyroidism

Elevated levels of the thyroid hormone increase metabolism and leads to hyperthyroidism. Women tend to have different symptoms with hyperthyroidism depending on if they have gone through menopause. Women who haven't gone through menopause may have symptoms such as:

- nervousness or anxiety
- weight loss

- heat intolerance
- sweating
- palpitations
- diarrhea
- tremors

Postmenopausal women may not have these typical symptoms and are more likely to have weight loss, constipation, loss of appetite, and mental or emotional changes.

Hyperthyroidism is detected by a low level of TSH in the blood. Since the thyroid is producing too much thyroid hormone, the body produces less TSH to try to decrease the thyroid hormone levels. Treatment is either through medications or surgery, depending on the cause of the hyperthyroidism. Hyperthyroidism can cause the heart to beat irregularly and also increases the risk of osteoporosis by accelerating the rate at which bone is broken down.

Testing for thyroid problems should be done in anyone with symptoms that suggest hypothyroidism or hyperthyroidism. Because older women have the highest chance of having these problems and because they may go unrecognized, some experts recommend that thyroid function be screened in older women on a regular basis.

FUTURE SCREENING TESTS

A number of tests are now available and are being evaluated to determine if they would be good screening tests in the future.

C-Reactive Protein

C-reactive protein or CRP is a blood test that indicates the presence of inflammation in the body. It is now believed that inflammation is the process behind most cardiovascular disease. In a study published in the *New England Journal of Medicine*, almost twenty-eight thousand women forty-five and older were studied over eight years. LDL cholesterol and CRP were measured and CRP was found to be a stronger predictor of future heart attacks and strokes than LDL.[50]

Of interest, the CRP and LDL tests tended to pick up different high risk groups. In other words, sometimes, the CRP would be normal and the LDL would be high or vice versa. Both groups of women were at higher risk for having a heart attack or stroke. Perhaps a combination of these tests will be a better way to identify those people who are higher risk because half of all heart attacks occur in people with no cholesterol problem.

However, there is controversy about the use of CRP as a screening test. It is unclear whether decreasing CRP will actually decrease the risk of heart disease. And the CRP values at which someone should be treated have yet to be determined. What's normal? What's too high? The Centers for Disease Control and Prevention and the American Heart Association are putting together guidelines on measuring and using CRP.

As noted, taking a baby aspirin (81mg) a day has been shown to reduce the chance of heart attack.[52] Perhaps it works by reducing inflammation and therefore CRP. Exercise has been shown to decrease CRP, even in the absence of weight loss.[53] Fat cells may contribute to elevated CRP so this may be yet another reason weight loss may be beneficial in protecting against cardiovascular disease.

Screening CT (Computed Tomography) Scans

Two new forms of screening are the electron-beam computed tomography (CT) and low-dose spiral computed tomography (CT) scans. These screening CT scans have recently been marketed directly to the public and are usually not covered by insurance. The fees generally range from $300 to $1,000.[54]

Electron-Beam CT Scan

The electron-beam CT is advertised as a screening test for undetected coronary artery disease. It does so by looking at the amount of calcium built up in the coronary arteries (the blood vessels that feed the heart). When these arteries are blocked, the blood supply to part of the heart is cut off, leading to a heart attack.

The test picks up about 80 percent of early heart disease, but 40 percent of the time it indicates an abnormality when there isn't one (a false positive result). The electron-beam CT is about as sensitive as other noninvasive tests for early heart disease but has a much higher false positive rate.[55] In a consensus statement from the American College of Cardiology and the American Heart Association, they did not currently recommend electron-beam CT for diagnosing obstructive coronary artery disease.[56]

Low-Dose Spiral CT Scan

Low-dose spiral CT scans have been advertised as a way to screen your whole body for cancers, tumors, aneurysms, osteoporosis, kidney and gallstones, spinal problems, and heart disease.[57] No rigorous data have been published on the use of CT scanning of the entire body to screen for cancers. No contrast agents are used, decreasing the ability of the scan to pick up small tumors in organs such as the liver, pancreas, and kidneys. For some organs, other tests such as ultrasound are better ways of evaluating them.

The biggest problem is that the scan would pick up something that would need to be evaluated further. This may involve further testing or invasive procedures which may be painful and potentially risky only to determine that the finding is benign. A normal test may lull some people into a false sense of security and they may feel they don't need to worry about cancer or heart disease.

Trials are underway to evaluate these technologies as to their usefulness. At this time, there is insufficient evidence to justify having screening CT scans done in women without any problems.

THE BOTTOM LINE

The most important thing is to have the screening tests done that are recommended by your physician and to be knowledgeable about other potential screening tests. The biggest problem is not having these tests done in the first place. A number of screening tests may be helpful to those of you who are at higher risk for certain problems. Discussing these other tests based on your personal and family medical history with your physician will help you determine if they would be beneficial to you. Communication of your concerns and discussion with your physician is of paramount importance. If you think that you need a test, be sure to discuss it with your physician. Though none of these tests is perfect, they are your best means to detect potential health problems early when you can do more to combat them.

AFTERWORD

Participating in the care of one's elderly parents and observing their death reminds us of our place in the universe, reinforcing the need to live fully, in the moment.

—Virginia Sharp Franz

F or many women, this time of transition is a wake-up call to improve their health. You start to realize that your body is not as forgiving of neglect or abuse as it once was. You also realize that your health, which you may have taken for granted, is something that needs to be cared for and protected. Unfortunately, many women do everything for everyone else first, putting their own needs last.

Now is the time to take control of your life and to take care of yourself. You know you have many things to do and at times they may seem overwhelming. Exercise, diet, time with your partner, time with family, and on and on it goes. So start with baby steps. Gradually introduce lifestyle changes that make sense to you. Can't even think about starting an exercise program? Start walking five minutes a day. Don't like the idea of no more sweets? Fine, just cut back.

You are more likely to stick with those gradual changes if they fit your lifestyle. If you radically change everything, you may be able to stick with it, but more likely you'll burn out and tire of all the changes, giving up and returning to your old ways. So start today taking small steps that together will add up to improved health in the long run. You're given only one body and it's up to you to care for it.

ADDITIONAL RESOURCES FOR WOMEN

*T*he Internet provides a wealth of information on a wide range of medical topics. Since there are no required standards, some information is inaccurate. It is best to consult sites developed by government agencies, nonprofits, and reputable companies. Here are several Web sites that provide a good starting point to find information about various health topics.

Women's Health Sites

Name	Address	Source	Highlights
National Women's Health Information Center	www.4woman.gov	Multiple government agencies and organizations	Web site and toll-free call center created by the U.S. Department of Health and Human Services to provide reliable health information for women.
North American Menopause Society	www.menopause.org	North American Menopause Society	Scientific nonprofit organization devoted to promoting women's health during midlife and beyond through an understanding of menopause. This site

			contains information on perimenopause, early menopause, menopause symptoms, and long-term health effects of estrogen loss, as well as a wide variety of therapies to enhance health.
The American College of Obstetricians and Gynecologists	www.acog.org	The American College of Obstetricians and Gynecologists	This is the Web site of the main organization for obstetricians and gynecologists in this country. There are a number of patient education materials and research articles related to women's health issues available on this site.
Foundation for Osteoporosis Research and Education	www.fore.org	Foundation for Osteoporosis Research and Education	Nonprofit resource center with information about osteoporosis, its diagnosis, prevention, and treatment.
National Osteoporosis Foundation	www.nof.org	National Osteoporosis Foundation	Nonprofit organization with comprehensive information about osteoporosis.
Women's Cancer Network	www.wcn.org	Gynecologic Cancer Foundation	Nonprofit organization that provides information that assists women who have developed cancer, as well as their families, to understand more about the disease, learn about treatment options, and gain access to new or experimental therapies about gynecologic and other cancers that affect women.
Planned Parenthood Federation of America	www.planned parenthood.org	Planned Parenthood Federation of America	Great source of information about birth control and sexually transmitted infections.

| American Social Health Association | www.ashastd.org | American Social Health Association | Nonprofit with information about sexually transmitted diseases and their prevention and treatment. |

General Health Information Sites

Name	Address	Source	Highlights
Health Finder	www.healthfinder.gov	Government agencies, nonprofit organizations, universities	A Web site that will lead you to reliable health information sources covering all aspects of medicine.
Health Topics A to Z	www.cdc.gov/health	Centers for Disease Control and Prevention	Health topics are arranged alphabetically and also by groups such as women's health, older adult health, and adolescent health.
Medline Plus	www.nlm.nih.gov/ medlineplus	National Institutes of Health and other reliable sources	Provides access to Medline, used to search scientific articles housed at the U.S. National Library of Medicine. This site also has directories for other reliable health information.
Family Doctor.org	www.familydoctor.org	American Academy of Family Physicians	Provides health information for the whole family, including resources on common medications.
MayoClinic.com	www.mayoclinic.com	Mayo Foundation for Medical Education and Research	Comprehensive and reliable resource for general health information.
Medem	www.medem.com	Member medical organizations	The medical library on this site includes patient information from all of the sponsoring medical organizations. This site

			also allows you to locate a physician where you live.
The Virtual Hospital	www.vh.org/	University of Iowa College of Medicine	A searchable medical resource for most common health problems.
InteliHealth	www.intelihealth.com	Harvard Medical School Faculty, NIH, and other health care organizations	Provides information about a variety of diseases and conditions. Has moderated chat rooms and discussion boards on a number of topics.
Laurus Health.com	www.LaurusHealth. com	Known public and private organizations, see list on site	Provides information about a variety of conditions and healthy living. Medline access is also available on this site.
Medscape Health from WebMD	www.medscape.com	Varies with topic selected	Provides access to medical news and reviews of journal articles for medical professionals but anyone who registers can have access to this information. There is an "Ask the Experts" section that answers frequently asked medical questions about a variety of conditions and problems.
Praxis.MD Practical Answers for Patients and Physicians	www.praxis.md	Clearly stated but varies with article	Information about a variety of medical topics can be found here. An interesting feature is a "Doctor Checklist" that contains illness-specific questions to answer before your visit to the doctor.

Prevention Sites

Name	Address	Source	Highlights
Harvard Center for Cancer Prevention	www.yourcancerrisk. Harvard.edu	Risk Index Working Group of Harvard University	You can calculate your risk for developing any of twelve different types of cancer and learn tips to prevent them.
The Official U.S. Government Site for People with Medicare	www.medicare.gov/ health/overview.asp	Governmental agencies	Provides information about Medicare benefits, publications, and Web sites with information that can help you stay healthy.
National Network for Immunization Information	www.immunization info.org	National Network for Immunization Information in partnership with the many medical organizations listed on the site	Provides up-to-date information about immunizations. Immunization schedules as well as state vaccine requirements are posted here.
American Lung Association	www.lungusa.org/ tobacco	American Lung Association	Information about lung health and illnesses can be found here. There is also information about the dangers of smoking and a free smoking cessation program.
National Safety Council	www.nsc.org	National Safety Council	Provides information on workplace, highway, community, and recreational safety to help raise awareness and to help reduce preventable injuries and death.

Nutrition and Activity Sites

Name	Address	Source	Highlights
American Dietetic Association	www.eatright.org	Clearly stated, but varies	An excellent site for information about nutrition

			depending upon area of the site you are visiting.	and food. Also provides advice on healthy eating habits and dieting.
Weight Loss and Control	www.niddk.nih.gov/ health/nutrit/nutrit.htm	National Institute of Diabetes & Digestive & Kidney Diseases		Good source of information about weight loss and control.
The Fitness Jumpsite	www.primusweb.com/ fitnesspartner/index. html	The Fitness Jumpsite		Provides information on exercise, diet, and weight management to help become more active and healthy. The Activity Calorie Calculator lets you put in your weight and number of minutes and it calculates the number of calories burned for different activities.
Milk Matters Education Campaign	www.nichd.nih.gov/ milk/milk.cfm	National Institute of Child Health and Human Development		Provides information on how to increase calcium consumption to strengthen bones.

Cancer Sites

Name	Address	Source	Highlights
National Cancer Institute	www.nci.nih.gov	PDQ database	Summaries of the most current information available on all aspects of cancer from prevention to alternative treatments.
Association of Online Cancer Resources	www.acor.org	Varies with selection	List of cancer-related support groups and Web sites.
Oncolink	www.oncolink.com	University of Pennsylvania Cancer Center	Source of information on a wide range of childhood and adult cancers, their treatment and clinical trials.

Heart Disease and Stroke Sites

Name	Address	Source	Highlights
National Heart, Lung, and Blood Institute	www.nhlbi.nih.gov	National Institutes of Health	Source of information about heart, lung, blood diseases, and sleeping disorders.
American Heart Association	www.americanheart.org	American Heart Association	An excellent source of information about heart disease, warning signs, risk factors, prevention, and treatment.
National Stroke Association	www.stroke.org	National Stroke Association	Information on stroke, its warning signs, prevention, and treatment is available on this site.
Cardiology Channel	www.cardiologychannel.com	Material developed and monitored by board-certified physicians	Provides basic information about different types of heart diseases.

Other Disease-Specific Sites

Name	Address	Source	Highlights
American Diabetes Association	www.diabetes.org	American Diabetes Association	Source of information about diabetes, its treatment, diet, and community resources.
An AIDS and HIV Information Resource—The Body	www.thebody.com	Varies with selection	Many articles on various aspects of HIV and AIDS are available.
HIV Institute	http://hivinsite.ucsf.edu/InSite.jsp	University of California San Francisco's Center for HIV Information	Comprehensive source of information about all aspects of HIV and AIDS.
National Institute of Mental Health	www.nimh.nih.gov/publicat/index.cfm	National Institute of Mental Health	Fact sheets on the symptoms and treatment options on a variety of mental health conditions can be found here.

Name	Address	Source	Highlights
National Strategy for Suicide Prevention	www.mentalhealth.org/suicideprevention/	Varies with section	A resource portal to learn about suicide and get prevention advice.
National Kidney Foundation	www.kidney.org	National Kidney Foundation	This site provides an opportunity to learn about kidney diseases. Information about kidney donation is also provided.
The Hormone Foundation	www.hormone.org	The Endocrine Society	Nonprofit organization that provides resources about hormone-related problems including diabetes, menopause, osteoporosis, obesity, and thyroid problems.
National Sleep Foundation	www.sleepfoundation.org	National Sleep Foundation	This site provides good advice about all types of sleep problems.
Endo-Online	www.endometriosisassn.org	Endometriosis Association	Site that provides information on endometriosis and its treatment.

Warning Web Sites

Name	Address	Source	Highlights
Quackwatch	www.quackwatch.com	Stephen Barrett, M.D.	An excellent site that provides informative articles and tips on how to spot and avoid medical fraud. Includes a listing and discussion of questionable medical practices and products.

Dietary Supplement Sites

Name	Address	Source	Highlights
Office of Dietary Supplements	http://dietary-supplements.info.nih.gov/	National Institutes of Health	Information is available on vitamins, minerals, botanical, and other dietary supplements.

Consumer Lab.com	www.consumerlab.com	Consumer Lab.com	This is an independent laboratory that tests and compares the stated ingredients in differing brands of vitamins, minerals, herbal products, other supplements, different foods, and personal care products. Because regulations for these sorts of products are not standardized, this provides more information about what's actually in these products.

Special Interest Sites

Name	Address	Source	Highlights
InfoAging.org	www.infoaging.org	American Federation of Aging Research	This site specializes in issues that face senior citizens. It provides information about diseases, the biology of aging, and healthy aging.
Black Health Online.com	www.blackhealth online.com	References given on all articles	This site gives information about diseases that commonly affect the Black community.
National Alliance for Hispanic Health	www.hispanichealth. org	National Alliance for Hispanic Health	Provides health information in both English and Spanish and is geared to the Hispanic community.
Asian American Health	www.nlm.nih.gov/ medlineplus/asian americanhealth.html	Varies with article selected	A resource of information about medical conditions that affect the Asian-American community.
Gay and Lesbian Medical Association	www.glma.org	Gay and Lesbian Medical Association	This site provides information on health concerns facing the gay and lesbian community.

Kids Health	www.kidshealth.org	KidsHealth.org	This site is devoted to the medical needs of children and adolescents. The site has areas geared toward children and teens as well as parents.
CYKE	www.cyke.com	Board-certified physicians	This site is dedicated to improving the emotional and physical health of children.
National Youth Violence Prevention Resource Center	www.safeyouth.org	All articles referenced	Source of information on prevention and intervention programs on youth violence and suicide. Warning signs to help parents and guardians recognize youth at risk are reviewed.
Antibiotic Guide	www.hopkins-abxguide.org	Johns Hopkins University Division of Infectious Diseases	You can search by drug or disease to learn what the experts would prescribe. Registration is required at no charge to access this wealth of information about antibiotics
RX Hope.com	www.rxhope.com	Rx Hope.com	The site provides information about assistance programs that are available for prescription medications.
Clarkhoward.com	www.clarkhoward.com	Clark Howard and staff	Advice for consumers on how spend less, save more, and avoid being cheated.

NOTES

CHAPTER 1. PERIMENOPAUSE TO MENOPAUSE: THE TRANSITION

1. Leon Speroff, Robert H. Glass, and Nathan G. Kase, *Clinical Gynecologic Endocrinology and Infertility*, 5th ed. (Baltimore, Md.: Williams and Wilkins, 1994), p. 583.

2. "Clinical Challenges of Perimenopause: Consensus Opinion of the North American Menopause Society," *Menopause* 7, no. 1 (2000): 5–13.

3. Howard Zacur et al., *Menopausal Health and Hormones: Enhancing Patient Management* (Johns Hopkins University School of Medicine: Quintiles Medical Communications, 2002), p. 4.

4. Ibid.

5. Ibid.

6. Speroff, Glass, and Kase, *Clinical Gynecologic Endocrinology and Infertility*, p. 587.

7. Ibid., p. 588.

CHAPTER 2. HOT FLASHES, NIGHT SWEATS, AND DRYNESS, OH MY!

1. "Clinical Challenges of Perimenopause: Consensus Opinion of the North American Menopause Society," *Menopause* 7, no. 1 (2000): 5–13.

2. F. Kronenberg, "Hot Flashes: Epidemiology and Physiology," *Annals of the New York Academy of Sciences* 592 (1990): 52–86.

3. Mary C. Martin et al., "Menopause without Symptoms: The Endocrinology of Menopause among Rural Mayan Indians," *American Journal of Obstetrics and Gynecology* 168, no. 8 (June 1993): 1839–45.

4. Barbara Kass-Annese, "Alternative Therapies for Menopause," *Clinical Obstetrics and Gynecology* 43, no. 1 (March 2000): 162–83.

5. Maura K. Whiteman et al., "Smoking, Body Mass, and Hot Flashes in Midlife Women," *Obstetrics and Gynecology* 101, no. 2 (February 2003): 264–72.

6. Ibid.

7. Margery L. S. Gass and Maida B. Taylor, "Alternatives for Women through Menopause," *American Journal of Obstetrics and Gynecology* 185, no. 2 (August 2001): S47–S56.

8. Susan R. Johnson, "Premenstrual Syndrome Therapy," *Clinical Obstetrics and Gynecology* 41, no. 2 (June 1998): 405–21.

9. Gass and Taylor, "Alternatives for Women through Menopause," pp. S47–S56.

10. Kishan J. Pandya et al., "Oral Clonidine in Postmenopausal Patients with Breast Cancer Experiencing Tamoxifen-Induced Hot Flashes: A University of Rochester Cancer Center Community Clinical Oncology Program Study," *Annals of Internal Medicine* 132, no. 10 (May 16, 2000): 788–93.

11. Gass and Taylor, "Alternatives for Women through Menopause," pp. S47–S56

12. *Menopause Core Curriculum Study Guide*, 2d ed. (Cleveland, Ohio: North American Menopause Society, 2002), p. 24.

13. Jacques Montplaisir et al., "Sleep in Menopause: Differential Effects of Two Forms of Hormone Replacement Therapy" *Menopause* 8, no. 1 (January 2001): 10–16.

14. Lynne Lamberg, "'Old and Gray and Full of Sleep'? Not Always," *Journal of the American Medical Association* 278, no. 16 (October 22–29, 1997): 1302–1304.

15. David J. Kupfer and Charles F. Reynolds III, "Current Concepts: Management of Insomnia," *New England Journal of Medicine* 336, no. 5 (January 30, 1997): 341–46.

16. I. Schiff et al., "Effects of Estrogen on Sleep and Psychological State of Hypogonadal Women," *Journal of the American Medical Association* 242 (1979): 2405–2407.

17. Kupfer and Reynolds III, "Current Concepts: Management of Insomnia," pp. 341–46.

18. Irina V. Zhdanova et al., "Melatonin Treatment for Age-Related Insomnia," *Journal of Clinical Endocrinology and Metabolism* 86, no. 10 (October 2001): 4727–30.

19. *Menopause Core Curriculum Study Guide*, p. 27.

20. Kathryn L. Burgio et al., "Behavioral vs. Drug Treatment for Urge Urinary Incontinence in Older Women: A Randomized Controlled Trial," *Journal of the American Medical Association* 280, no. 23 (December 16, 1998): 1995–2000.

21. Kathryn L. Burgio et al., "Behavioral Training with and without Biofeedback in the Treatment of Urge Incontinence in Older Women: A Randomized Controlled Trial," *Journal of the American Medical Association* 288, no. 18 (November 13, 2002): 2293–99.

22. James Malone-Lee et al., "Tolterodine: Superior Tolerability Than and Comparable Efficacy to Oxybutynin in Individuals 50 Years Old or Older with Overactive Bladder: A Randomized Controlled Trial," *Journal of Urology* 165, no. 5 (May 2001): 1452–56.

23. Peter L. Dwyer and Mary O'Reilly, "Recurrent Urinary Tract Infection in the Female," *Current Opinion in Obstetrics and Gynecology* 14, no. 5 (October 2002): 537–43.

24. Janet Rose Osuch, "Breast Health and Disease over a Lifetime," *Clinical Obstetrics and Gynecology* 45, no. 4 (December 2002): 1140–61.

25. Ibid.

26. Antonio V. Millet and Frederick M. Dirbas, "Clinical Management of Breast Pain: A Review," *Obstetrical and Gynecological Survey* 57, no. 7 (July 2002): 451–61.

27. Ibid.

28. Naomi Breslau and Birthe Krogh Rasmussen, "The Impact of Migraines: Epidemiology, Risk Factors, and Co-morbidities," *Neurology* 56, no. 6 (March 2001): S4–S12.

29. Stephen D. Silberstein, "Headache and Female Hormones: What You Need to Know," *Current Opinion in Neurology* 14, no. 3 (June 2001): 323–33.

30. Breslau and Rasmussen "The Impact of Migraines: Epidemiology, Risk factors, and Co-morbidities," pp. S4–S12.

31. K. M. A. Welch, "A 47-Year-Old Woman with Tension-Type Headaches," *Journal of the American Medical Association* 286, no. 8 (August 22–29, 2001): 960–66.

32. B. K. Rasmussen, "Migraine and Tension-Type Headache in a General Population: Precipitating Factors, Female Hormones, Sleep Pattern, and Relation to Lifestyle," *Pain* 53, no. 1 (April 1993): 65–72.

33. Ivy Fettes, "Migraine in the Menopause," *Neurology* 54, no. 4, supp. 1 (September 1999): S29–S33.

34. D. M. Jacobs et al., "Cognitive Function in Nondemented Older Women Who Took Estrogen after Menopause," *Neurology* 50, no. 20 (February 1998): 368–73; Susan M. Resnick, Jeffrey E. Metter, and Alan B. Zonderman, "Estrogen Replacement Therapy and Longitudinal Decline in Visual Memory: A Possible Protective Effect?" *Neurology* 49, no. 6 (December 1997): 1491–97.

35. Kenneth J. Mukamal et al., "Prospective Study of Alcohol Consumption and Risk of Dementia in Older Adults," *Journal of the American Medical Associ-*

ation 289, no. 11 (March 19, 2003): 1405–13; Gary W. Small, "What We Need to Know about Age Related Memory Loss," *British Medical Journal* 324, no. 7352 (June 22, 2002): 1502–1505.

36. Ibid.

CHAPTER 3. MY PERIODS HAVE CHANGED. SHOULD I WORRY?

1. Andrew Prentice, "Fortnightly Review: Medical Management of Menorrhagia," *British Medical Journal* 319, no. 7221 (November 20, 1999): 1343–45.

2. Charles M. March, "Bleeding Problems and Treatment," *Clinical Obstetrics and Gynecology* 41, no. 4 (December 1998): 928–39.

3. Alexander C. Lai et al., "Sexual Dysfunction after Uterine Artery Embolization," *Journal of Vascular and Interventional Radiology* 11, no. 6 (June 2000): 755–58.

4. R. J. Kurman et al., "The Behavior of Endometrial Hyperplasia: A Long-Term Study of 'Untreated' Hyperplasia in 170 Patients," *Cancer* 56 (1985): 403.

5. Ibid.

6. "What Are the Key Statistics for Endometrial Cancer?" *American Cancer Society* [online], www.cancer.org [May 12, 2003].

7. March, "Bleeding Problems and Treatment," pp. 928–39.

CHAPTER 4. WHAT'S WITH MY MOODS?

1. Lorraine Dennerstein et al., "Factors Contributing to Positive Mood during the Menopausal Transition," *Journal of Nervous and Mental Disease* 189, no. 2 (February 2001): 84–89.

2. Marilyn I. Korzekwa and Meir Steiner, "Premenstrual Syndromes," *Clinical Obstetrics and Gynecology* 40, no. 3 (September 1997): 564–76.

3. Ibid.

4. Barbara L. Parry, "A 45-Year-Old Woman with Premenstrual Dysphoric Disorder," *Journal of the American Medical Association* 281, no. 4 (January 27, 1999): 368–73.

5. Korzekwa and Steiner, "Premenstrual Syndromes," pp. 564–76.

6. Parry, "A 45-Year-Old Woman with Premenstrual Dysphoric Disorder," pp. 368–73.

7. Susan R. Johnson, "Premenstrual Syndrome Therapy," *Clinical Obstetrics and Gynecology* 41, no. 2 (June 1998): 405–21.

8. Ibid.

9. Clare Stevinson and Edzard Ernst, "Complementary/Alternative Thera-

pies for Premenstrual Syndrome: A Systemic Review of Randomized Controlled trials," *American Journal of Obstetrics and Gynecology* 185, no. 1 (July 2001): 227–35.

10. Johnson, "Premenstrual Syndrome Therapy," pp. 405–21.

11. Ibid.

12. Katrina Wyatt et al., "Efficacy of Progesterone and Progestogens in Management of Premenstrual Syndrome: Systemic Review," *British Medical Journal* 323, no. 7316 (October 6, 2001): 776–80.

13. *2003 Compendium of Selected Publications* (Washington, D.C.: American College of Obstetricians and Gynecologists, 2003), p. 542.

14. Johnson, "Premenstrual Syndrome Therapy," pp. 405–21.

15. Ibid.

16. Jan P. Vleck and Sarab M. Safranek, "What Medications Are Effective for Treating Symptoms of Premenstrual Syndrome (PMS)?" *Journal of Family Practice* 51, no. 10 (October 2002): 894; Teri Pearlstein, "Selective Serotonin Reuptake Inhibitors for Premenstrual Dysphoric Disorder: The Emerging Gold Standard?" *Drugs* 62, no. 13 (2002): 1869–85.

17. Pearlstein, "Selective Serotonin Reuptake Inhibitors."

18. Johnson, "Premenstrual Syndrome Therapy," pp. 405–21.

19. Ellen W. Freeman et al., "A Double-Blind Trial of Oral Progesterone, Alprazolam, and Placebo in Treatment of Severe Premenstrual Syndrome," *Journal of the American Medical Association* 274, no. 1 (July 5, 1995): 51–57.

20. Johnson, "Premenstrual Syndrome Therapy," pp. 405–21.

21. Ibid.

22. Sheryl A. Kingsberg, "Reproductive Senescence and Depression Revisited (Again)," *Menopause* 9, no. 6 (November 2002): 389–91.

23. "Let's Talk Facts about Depression," *American Psychiatric Association* [online], www.psych.org/public_info/depression.cfm [May 5, 2003].

24. "Psychiatric Medications," *American Psychiatric Association* [online], http://www.psych.org/public_info/medication.cfm#antidepressants [May 5, 2003].

25. Peter J. Schmidt et al., "Estrogen Replacement in Perimenopause-Related Depression: A Preliminary Report," *American Journal of Obstetrics and Gynecology* 183, no. 2 (August 2000): 414–20; Claudio de Novaes Soares et al., "Efficacy of Estradiol for the Treatment of Depressive Disorders in Perimenopausal Women: A Double-Blind, Randomized, Placebo-Controlled Trial," *Archives of General Psychiatry* 58, no. 6 (June 2001): 529–34.

26. Leon Speroff, *Managing Menopause: A Clinician's Guidebook* (Montvale, N.J.: Thomson Medical Economics, 2002), p. 55.

27. M. Kull, "The Relationships between Physical Activity, Health Status, and Psychological Well-Being of Fertility-Aged Women," *Scandinavian Journal of Medicine and Science in Sports* 12, no. 4 (August 2002): 241–47.

CHAPTER 5. PACKING ON THE POUNDS

1. Katherine M. Flegal, "Prevalence and Trends in Obesity among U.S. Adults, 1999–2000," *Journal of the American Medical Association* 288, no. 14 (October 9, 2002): 1723–27.

2. Vivian M. Dickerson, "Focus on Primary Care: Evaluation, Management, and Treatment of Obesity in Women," *Obstetrical and Gynecological Survey* 56, no. 10 (2001): 650–63.

3. *Clinical Guidelines on the Identification, Evaluation, and Treatment of Overweight and Obesity in Adults,* NIH Publication No. 98-4083 (Bethesda, Md.: National Institutes of Health, September 1998), pp. 12–18.

4. Anna Peeters et al., "Obesity in Adulthood and Its Consequences for Life Expectancy: A Life-Table Analysis," *Annals of Internal Medicine* 138, no. 1 (January 7, 2003): 24–32.

5. Eugenia E. Calle et al., "Overweight, Obesity, and Mortality from Cancer in a Prospectively Studied Cohort of U.S. Adults," *New England Journal of Medicine* 348, no. 17 (April 24, 2003): 1625–38.

6. George S. Roth et al., "Caloric Restriction in Primates and Relevance to Humans," *Annals of the New York Academy of Sciences* 928 (2001): 305–15.

7. John M. Jakicic et al., "Appropriate Intervention Strategies for Weight Loss and Prevention of Weight Regain for Adults," *Medicine and Science in Sports and Exercise* 33, no. 12 (December 2001): 2145–56.

8. *The Practical Guide: Identification, Evaluation, and Treatment of Overweight and Obesity in Adults,* NIH Publication Number 00-4084 (Bethesda, Md.: National Institutes of Health; National Heart, Lung, and Blood Institute; North American Association for the Study of Obesity, October 2000), p. 9.

9. J. C. Lovejoy, "The Influence of Sex Hormones on Obesity across the Female Life Span," *Journal of Woman's Health* 7, no. 10 (December 1998): 1247–56.

10. Arne Astrup, "Physical Activity and Weight Gain and Fat Distribution Changes with Menopause: Current Evidence and Research Issues," *Medicine and Science in Sports and Exercise* 31, no. 11, suppl. 1 (November 1999): S564; Eric T. Poehlman, "Menopause, Energy Expenditure, and Body Composition," *Acta Obstetricia et Gynecologica Scandanavica* 81, no. 7 (July 2002): 603–11.

11. Eric T. Poehlman et al., "Changes in Energy Balance and Body Composition at Menopause: A Controlled Longitudinal Study," *Annals of Internal Medicine* 123, no. 9 (November 1, 1995): 673–75.

12. S. L. Crawford et al., "A Longitudinal Study of Weight and the Menopause Transition: Results from the Massachusetts Women's Health Study," *Menopause* 7, no. 2 (March–April 2000): 96–104.

13. Samara Joy Nielsen and Barry M. Popkin, "Patterns and Trends in Food Portion Sizes, 1977–1998," *Journal of the American Medical Association* 289, no. 4 (January 22/29 2003): 450–53.

14. Poehlman et al., "Changes in Energy Balance and Body Composition at Menopause: A Controlled Longitudinal Study," pp. 673–75.

15. Judith Korner and Louis J. Aronne, "The Emerging Science of Body Weight Regulation and Its Impact on Obesity Treatment," *Journal of Clinical Investigation* 111, no. 5 (March 2003): 565–70.

16. Todd M. Sheperd, "Effective Management of Obesity," *Journal of Family Practice* 52, no. 1 (January 2003): 34–42.

17. Frank Hu et al., "Trans-fatty Acids and Coronary Heart Disease," *New England Journal of Medicine* 340 (1999): 1994–98.

18. Tom A. B. Sanders, "High- versus Low-fat Diets in Human Diseases," *Current Opinion in Clinical Nutrition and Metabolic Care* 6, no. 2 (March 2003): 151–55.

19. Martha Clare Morris et al., "Dietary Fats and the Risk of Incident Alzheimer Disease," *Archives of Neurology* 60, no. 2 (February 2003): 194–200.

20. David S. Ludwig, "The Glycemic Index: Physiological Mechanisms Relating to Obesity, Diabetes, and Cardiovascular Disease," *Journal of the American Medical Association* 287, no. 18 (May 8, 2002): 2414–23.

21. "The Truth about Dieting," *Consumer Reports* 67, no. 6 (June 2002): 26–31.

22. Jakicic et al., "Appropriate Intervention Strategies for Weight Loss and Prevention of Weight Regain for Adults," pp. 2145–56.

23. Ibid.

24. Paul G. Shekelle et al., "Efficacy and Safety of Ephedra and Ephedrine for Weight Loss and Athletic Performance: A Meta-analysis," *Journal of the American Medical Association* 289, no. 12 (March 26, 2003): 1537–45; Christine A. Haller and Neal L. Benowitz, "Adverse Cardiovascular and Central Nervous System Events Associated with Dietary Supplements Containing Ephedra Alkaloids," *New England Journal of Medicine* 343, no. 25 (December 21, 2000): 1833–38.

25. Joya T. Favreau et al., "Severe Hepatotoxicity Associated with the Dietary Supplement LipoKinetix," *Annals of Internal Medicine* 136, no. 8 (April 16, 2002): 590–95.

CHAPTER 6. NOT IN THE MOOD

1. John Gray, *Men Are from Mars, Women Are from Venus: A Practical Guide for Improving Communication and Getting What You Want in Your Relationships* (New York: HarperCollins Publishers, 1992).

2. L. Dennerstein et al., "Sexuality and the Menopause," *Psychosom Obstet Gynaecol* 15 (1994): 59–66.

3. Tiffany M. Field et al., "Tactile/Kinesthetic Stimulation Effects on Preterm Neonates," *Pediatrics* 77, no. 5 (May 1986): 654–58.

4. Tiffany M. Field, "Massage Therapy Effects," *American Psychologist* 53, no. 12 (December 1998): 1270–81.

5. Cindy M. Meston and Penny F. Frohlich, "The Neurobiology of Sexual Function," *Archives of General Psychiatry* 57, no. 11 (November 2000): 1012–30.

6. Aristotelis G. Anastasiadis et al., "Hormonal Factors in Female Sexual Dysfunction," *Current Opinion in Urology* 12, no. 6 (November 2002): 503–507.

7. Ibid.

8. Meston and Frohlich, "The Neurobiology of Sexual Function," pp. 1012–30.

9. Ibid.

10. Anastasiadis et al., "Hormonal Factors in Female Sexual Dysfunction," pp. 503–507.

11. Ibid.

12. Rogerio A. Lobo, "Androgens in Postmenopausal Women: Production, Possible Role, and Replacement Options," *Obstetrical and Gynecological Survey* 56, no. 6 (June 2001): 361–76.

13. Xavier Bosch, "Please Don't Pass the Paella: Eating Disorders Upset Spain," *Journal of the American Medical Association* 283, no. 11 (March 15, 2000): 1405–10.

14. Linda Bernhard, "Sexuality and Sexual Health Care for Women," *Clinical Obstetrics and Gynecology* 45, no. 4 (December 2002): 1089–98.

15. A. Hordern, "Intimacy and Sexuality for the Woman with Breast Cancer," *Cancer Nursing* 23, no. 3 (June 2000): 230–36.

16. Meston and Frohlich, "The Neurobiology of Sexual Function," pp. 1012–30.

17. Julia R. Heiman and Cindy M. Meston, "Evaluating Sexual Dysfunction in Women," *Clinical Obstetrics and Gynecology* 40, no. 3 (September 1997): 616–29.

CHAPTER 7. I CAN'T BE PREGNANT . . .

1. Andrew Kaunitz, "Oral Contraceptive Use in Perimenopause," *American Journal of Obstetrics and Gynecology* 85, no. 2, supp. (August 2001): S32–S37.

2. Carolyn Westhoff, "Contraception at Age 35 Years and Older," *Clinical Obstetrics and Gynecology* 41, no. 4 (December 1998): 951–57.

3. Leon Speroff and Philip Darney, *A Clinical Guide for Contraception* (Baltimore, Md.: Williams & Wilkins, 1996), p. 5.

4. Ibid.

5. Ibid.

6. Westhoff, "Contraception at Age 35 Years and Older," p. 953.

7. Patricia J. Sulak and Arthur F. Haney, "Unwanted Pregnancies: Under-

standing Contraceptive Use and Benefits in Adolescents and Older Women," *American Journal of Obstetrics and Gynecology* 168, no. 6S (June 1993): 2042–48.

8. Ibid.

9. Westhoff, "Contraception at Age 35 Years and Older," p. 953.

10. Ronald T. Burkman et al., "Current Perspectives on Oral Contraceptive Use," *American Journal of Obstetrics and Gynecology* 185, no. 2, supp. (August 2001): S4–S12.

11. Polly A. Marchbanks et al., "Oral Contraceptives and the Risk of Breast Cancer," *New England Journal of Medicine* 346, no. 26 (June 27, 2002): 2025–32.

12. Burkman, "Current Perspectives on Oral Contraceptive Use," S4–S12.

13. Speroff and Darney, *A Clinical Guide for Contraception.*

14. Ibid.

15. Victoria L. Holt, Kara L. Cushing-Haugen, and Janet R. Daling, "Body Weight and Risk of Oral Contraceptive Failure," *Obstetrics and Gynecology* 99, no. 5 (May 2002): 820–27.

16. Speroff and Darney, *A Clinical Guide for Contraception*, p. 78.

17. Ibid.

18. Miriam Zieman et al., "Contraceptive Efficacy and Cycle Control with the Ortho Evra Transdermal System: The Analysis of Pooled Data," *Fertility and Sterility* 77, no. 2, supp. (February 2002): S13–S18.

19. Speroff and Darney, *A Clinical Guide for Contraception*, p. 178.

20. Ibid., p. 179.

21. Ibid., p. 184.

22. Ibid., p. 200.

23. Ibid., p. 330.

24. Brian Cox et al., "Vasectomy and Risk of Prostate Cancer," *Journal of the American Medical Association* 287, no. 23 (June 19, 2002): 3110–15.

25. Matthew A. Cohen and Mark V. Sauer, "Fertility in Perimenopausal Women," *Clinical Obstetrics and Gynecology* 41, no. 4 (December 1998): 958–65.

26. William N. Spellacy et al., "Pregnancy after 40 Years of Age," *Obstetrics and Gynecology* 68 (1986): 452–54.

CHAPTER 8. SINGLE AGAIN AND AVOIDING SEXUALLY TRANSMITTED DISEASES

1. "Tracking the Hidden Epidemics 2000: Trends in STDs in the United States," *Centers for Disease Control and Prevention* [online], www.cdc.gov/nchstp/od/news/RevBrochure1pdftoc.htm [May 5, 2003].

2. Ibid.

3. Ibid.

4. Ibid.

5. "Genital Herpes Fact Sheet," *CDC Division of Sexually Transmitted Diseases* [online], http://www.cdc.gov/nchstp/dstd/Fact_Sheets/facts_Genital_Herpes. htm [May 5, 2003].

6. "Genital HPV Infection," *CDC Division of Sexually Transmitted Diseases* [online], http://www.cdc.gov/nchstp/dstd/Fact_Sheets/FactsHPV.htm [May 5, 2003].

7. "Cancer Facts and Figures 2001," *American Cancer Society* [online], www.cancer.org [May 9, 2003].

8. Pamela J. Paley, "Screening for the Major Malignancies Affecting Women: Current Guidelines," *American Journal of Obstetrics and Gynecology* 184 (April 2001): 1025.

9. *2003 Compendium of Selected Publications* (Washington, D.C.: American College of Obstetricians and Gynecologists, 2003), p. 689.

10. Ibid.

11. David E. Cohn and Thomas J. Herzog, "New Innovations in Cervical Cancer Screening," *Clinical Obstetrics and Gynecology* 44, no. 3 (September 2001): 538–49.

12. Paley, "Screening for the Major Malignancies Affecting Women: Current Guidelines," pp. 1021–30.

13. *2003 Compendium of Selected Publications*, p. 689.

14. "Tracking the Hidden Epidemics 2000: Trends in STDs in the United States," *Centers for Disease Control and Prevention* [online], www.cdc.gov/ nchstp/od/news/RevBrochure1pdftoc.htm [May 5, 2003].

15. Ibid.

16. "Viral Hepatitis B Fact Sheet," *CDC National Center for Infectious Diseases* [online], http://www.cdc.gov/ncidod/diseases/hepatitis/b/fact.htm [May 5, 2003].

17. Ibid.

18. Ibid.

19. Ibid.

20. "Tracking the Hidden Epidemics 2000: Trends in STDs in the United States."

21. "Update: AIDS—United States, 2000," *Morbidity and Mortality Weekly Report* 51, no. 27 (July 12, 2002): 592–95.

22. "HIV/AIDS Surveillance Report: U.S. HIV and AIDS Cases Reported through December 2001," *Centers for Disease Control and Prevention* [online], http://www.cdc.gov/hiv/stats/hasr1302/table7.htm [May 5, 2003].

23. Dennis H. Osmond, "Sexual Transmission of HIV," *HIV InSite Knowledge Base Chapter* [online], http://hivinsite.ucsf.edu [May 6, 2003].

24. Erica Weir, "Drug-Facilitated Date Rape," *Canadian Medical Association Journal* 165, no. 1 (July 10, 2001): 80.

25. Ibid.

26. "Forensics," *Drink Safe Technology* [online], www.drinksafetech.com [May 6, 2003].

CHAPTER 9. HORMONES:
THE GOOD, THE BAD, AND THE UGLY

1. Wulf H. Utian et al., "Relief of Vasomotor Symptoms and Vaginal Atrophy with Lower Doses of Conjugated Equine Estrogens and Medroxyprogesterone Acetate," *Fertility and Sterility* 75, no. 6 (June 2001): 1065–79.

2. Paivi Polo-Kantola et al., "When Does Estrogen Replacement Therapy Improve Sleep Quality?" *American Journal of Obstetrics and Gynecology* 178, no. 5 (May 1998): 1002–1009.

3. Philip M. Sarrel, "Sexuality and Menopause," *Obstetrics and Gynecology* 75, no. 4, supp. (April 1990): 26S.

4. Bjaren C. Eriksen, "A Randomized, Open, Parallel-Group Study on the Preventive Effect of an Estradiol-Releasing Vaginal Ring (Estring) on Recurrent Urinary Tract Infections in Postmenopausal Women," *American Journal of Obstetrics and Gynecology* 180, no. 5 (May 1999): 1072–79.

5. J. Andrew Fantl et al., "Estrogen Therapy in the Management of Urinary Incontinence in Postmenopausal Women: A Meta-analysis. First Report of the Hormones and Urogenital Therapy Committee," *Obstetrics and Gynecology* 83, no. 1 (January 1994): 12–18.

6. D. M. Jacobs et al., "Cognitive Function in Nondemented Older Women Who Took Estrogen after Menopause," *Neurology* 50, no. 20 (February 1998): 368–73.

7. Claudio de Novaes Soares et al., "Efficacy of Estradiol for the Treatment of Depressive Disorders in Perimenopausal Women: A Double-Blind, Randomized, Placebo-Controlled Trial," *Archives of General Psychiatry* 58, no. 6 (June 2001): 529–34.

8. Orhan Bukulmez et al., "Short-Term Effects of Three Continuous Hormone Replacement Therapy Regimens on Platelet Tritiated Imipramine Binding and Mood Scores: A Prospective Randomized Trial," *Fertility and Sterility* 75, no. 4 (April 2001): 737–43.

9. Peter P. Zandi et al., "Hormone Replacement Therapy and Incidence of Alzheimer Disease in Older Women: The Cache County Study," *Journal of the American Medical Association* 288, no. 17 (November 6, 2002): 2123–29.

10. V. W. Henderson et al., "Estrogen for Alzheimer's Disease in Women: Randomized, Double-Blind, Placebo-Controlled Trial," *Neurology* 54, no. 2 (January 25, 2000): 295–301.

11. Tord Naessen et al., "Better Postural Balance in Elderly Women Receiving Estrogens," *American Journal of Obstetrics and Gynecology* 177, no. 2 (August 1997): 412–16.

12. Roberto Civitelli et al., "Alveolar and Postcranial Bone Density in Postmenopausal Women Receiving Hormone/Estrogen Replacement Therapy," *Archives of Internal Medicine* 162, no. 12 (June 24, 2002): 1409–15.

13. Jacques E. Rossouw et al., "Risks and Benefits of Estrogen Plus Progestin in Healthy Postmenopausal Women: Principal Results from the Women's Health Initiative Randomized Controlled Trial," *Journal of the American Medical Association* 288, no. 3 (July 17, 2002): 321–33.

14. Laura B. Dunn et al., "Does Estrogen Prevent Skin Aging?: Results from the First National Health and Nutrition Examination Survey (NHANES I)," *Archives of Dermatology* 133, no. 3 (March 1997): 339–42.

15. "Hormone Replacement Study a Shock to the Medical System, July 10, 2002," *New York Times* [online], www.nytimes.com [May 15, 2003].

16. "Amended Report from the NAMS Advisory Panel on Postmenopausal Hormone Therapy," *Menopause* 10, no. 1 (January 2003): 6–12.

17. Leon Speroff, Robert H. Glass, and Nathan G. Kase, *Clinical Gynecologic Endocrinology and Infertility*, 5th ed. (Baltimore, Md.: Williams and Wilkins, 1994), p. 618.

18. Akihiko Wakatsuki et al., "Different Effects of Oral Conjugated Equine Estrogen and Transdermal Estrogen Replacement Therapy on Size and Oxidative Susceptibility of Low-Density Lipoprotein Particles in Postmenopausal Women," *Circulation* 106, no. 14 (October 1, 2002): 1771–76.

19. Andrea Decensi et al., "Effect of Transdermal Estradiol and Oral Conjugated Estrogen on C-Reactive Protein in Retinoid-Placebo Trial in Healthy Women," *Circulation* 106, no. 10 (September 3, 2002): 1224–28.

20. Maida Taylor, "Unconventional Estrogens: Estriol, Biest, and Triest," *Clinical Obstetrics and Gynecology* 44, no. 4 (December 2001): 864–79.

21. Ibid.

22. Peter G. Rose, "Medical Progress: Endometrial Carcinoma," *New England Journal of Medicine* 335, no. 9 (August 29, 1996): 640–49.

23. "Role of Progesterone in Hormone Therapy for Postmenopausal Women: Position Statement of the North American Menopause Society," *Menopause* 10, no. 2 (2003): 113–32.

24. Barry G. Wren et al., "Transdermal Progesterone and Its Effect on Vasomotor Symptoms, Blood Lipid Levels, Bone Metabolic Markers, Moods, and Quality of Life for Postmenopausal Women," *Menopause* 10, no. 1 (January 2003): 13–18.

25. Aristotelis G. Anastasiadis et al., "Hormonal Factors in Female Sexual Dysfunction," *Current Opinion in Urology* 12, no. 6 (November 2002): 503–507.

26. Ma Clara Padero, Shalender Bhasin, and Theodore C. Friedman, "Androgen Supplementation in Older Women: Too Much Hype, Not Enough Data," *Journal of the American Geriatrics Society* 50, no. 6 (June 2002): 1131–40.

27. Rogerio A. Lobo, "Androgens in Postmenopausal Women: Production, Possible Role, and Replacement Options," *Obstetrical and Gynecological Survey* 56, no. 6 (June 2001): 361–76.

28. Ibid.

29. Omid Khorram, "Androgens in Women," *Clinical Obstetrics and Gynecology* 44, no. 4 (December 2001): 880–92.

30. Lawrence B. Riggs and Lynn C. Hartmann, "Drug Therapy: Selective Estrogen-Receptor Modulators—Mechanisms of Action and Application to Clinical Practice," *New England Journal of Medicine* 348, no. 7 (February 13, 2003): 618–29.

31. Ibid., pp. 864–79.

CHAPTER 10. NATURAL REMEDIES: WHAT THEY DON'T TELL YOU

1. "What Is Complementary and Alternative Medicine (CAM)?" *National Center for Complementary and Alternative Medicine* [online], http://nccam.nih.gov/health/whatiscam/ [May 13, 2003].

2. "Use of Botanicals for Management of Menopausal Symptoms," *ACOG Practice Bulletin* 28 (June 2001): 2.

3. Ibid.

4. "Regulations on Statements Made for Dietary Supplements Concerning the Effect of the Product on the Structure or Function of the Body; Final Rule," *U.S. Food and Drug Administration Center for Food Safety and Applied Nutrition* [online], http://www.cfsan.fda.gov/~lrd/fr000106.html [May 13, 2003].

5. "Overview of Dietary Supplements," *U. S. Food and Drug Administration Center for Food Safety and Applied Nutrition* http://www.cfsan.fda.gov/~dms/ds-oview.html [May 13, 2003].

6. "Kava: A Supplement to Avoid," *Consumer Report* 68, no. 3 (March 2003).

7. Bill J. Gurley, Stephanie F. Gardner, and Martha A. Hubbard, "Content versus Label Claims in Ephedra-Containing Dietary Supplements," *American Journal of Health-Systems Pharmacy* 57 (May 15, 2000): 963–69.

8. Donald M. Marcus and Arthur P. Grollman, "Botanical Medicines—The Need for New Regulations," *New England Journal of Medicine* 347, no. 25 (December 19, 2002): 2073–76.

9. Ibid.

10. "Use of Botanicals for Management of Menopausal Symptoms," p. 4.

11. Judith S. Jacobson et al., "Randomized Trial of Black Cohosh for the Treatment of Hot Flashes among Women with a History of Breast Cancer," *Journal of Clinical Oncology* 19 (May 15, 2001): 2739–45.

12. Hussein R. Chenoy et al., "Effect of Oral Gamolenic Acid from Evening Primrose Oil on Menopausal Flushing," *British Medical Journal* 308 (February 19, 1994): 501–503.

13. Antonio V. Millet and Frederick M. Dirbas, "Clinical Management of Breast Pain: A Review," *Obstetrical and Gynecological Survey* 57, no. 7 (July 2002): 451–61.

14. Maida Taylor, "Botanicals: Medicines and Menopause," *Clinical Obstetrics and Gynecology* 44, no. 4 (December 2001): 853–63.

15. "Use of Botanicals for Management of Menopausal Symptoms," p. 4.

16. Paula Amato et al., "Estrogenic Activity of Herbs Commonly Used as Remedies for Menopausal Symptoms," *Menopause* 9, no. 2 (March 2002): 145–50.

17. Taylor, "Botanicals," pp. 853–63.

18. R. J. Baber et al., "Randomized Placebo-Controlled Trial of an Isoflavone Supplement and Menopausal Symptoms," *Climacteric* 2, no. 2 (June 1999): 85–92.

19. Adriane Fugh-Berman and Fredi Kronenberg, "Red Clover (*Trifolium pratense*) for Menopausal Women: Current State of Knowledge," *Menopause* 8, no. 5 (September 2001): 333–37.

20. Taylor, "Botanicals," pp. 853–63.

21. "Role of Progesterone in Hormone Therapy for Postmenopausal Women: Position Statement of the North American Menopause Society," *Menopause* 10, no. 2 (2003): 113–32.

22. Taylor, "Botanicals," pp. 853–63.

23. Lucinda G. Miller, "Herbal Medicinals: Selected Clinical Considerations Focusing on Known or Potential Drug-Herb Interactions," *Archives of Internal Medicine* 158, no. 20 (November 9, 1998): 2200–11.

24. Taylor, "Botanicals," pp. 853–63.

25. Amato et al., "Estrogenic Activity of Herbs," pp. 145–50.

26. Edzard Ernst, "The Risk-Benefit Profile of Commonly Used Herbal Therapies: Ginkgo, St. John's Wort, Ginseng, Echinacea, Saw Palmetto, and Kava," *Annals of Internal Medicine* 136, no. 1 (January 1, 2002): 42–53.

27. R. Schellenberg, "Treatment for the Premenstrual Syndrome with Agnus castus Fruit Extract: Prospective, Randomised, Placebo Controlled Study," *British Medical Journal* 322, no. 7279 (January 20, 2001): 134–37.

28. Clare Stevinson and Edzard Ernst, "Complementary/Alternative Therapies for Premenstrual Syndrome: A Systemic Review of Randomized Controlled Trials," *American Journal of Obstetrics and Gynecology* 185, no. 1 (July 2001): 227–35.

29. Lori Russell et al., "Phytoestrogens: A Viable Option?" *American Journal of Medical Sciences* 324, no. 4 (October 2002): 185–88.

30. A. L. Edralin et al., "Flaxseed Improves Lipid Profile without Altering Biomarkers of Bone Metabolism in Postmenopausal Women," *Journal of Clinical Endocrinoogy and Metababolism* 87 (2002): 1527–32.

31. Evelyne D. Faure, Philippe Chantre, and Pierre Mares, "Effects of a Standardized Soy Extract on Hot Flushes: A Multicenter, Double-Blind, Randomized, Placebo-Controlled Study," *Menopause* 9, no. 5 (September 2002): 329–34.

32. A. A. Ewies, "A Comprehensive Approach to the Menopause: So Far, One Size Should Fit All," *Obstetrical and Gynecological Survey* 56, no. 10 (October 2001): 642–49.

33. F. Kronenberg and A. Fugh-Berman, "Soy and Hot Flashes," *Alternative Therapies in Women's Health* 4, no. 9 (September 2002): 68–71.

34. Cheri L. Van Patten et al., "Effect of Soy Phytoestrogens on Hot Flashes in Postmenopausal Women with Breast Cancer: A Randomized, Controlled Clinical Trial," *Journal of Clinical Oncology* 20, no. 6 (March 15, 2002): 1449–55.

35. "Use of Botanicals for Management of Menopausal Symptoms," p. 7.

36. Ernst, "The Risk-Benefit Profile of Commonly Used Herbal Therapies," pp. 42–53.

37. Miller, "Herbal Medicinals," pp. 2200–11.

38. Ernst, "The Risk-Benefit Profile of Commonly Used Herbal Therapies," pp. 42–53.

39. Ibid.

40. Mitra Assemi, "Herbs Affecting the Central Nervous System: Ginko, Kava, St. John's Wort, and Valerian," *Clinical Obstetrics and Gynecology* 44, no. 4 (December 2001): 824–35.

41. Barbara Kass-Annese, "Alternative Therapies for Menopause," *Clinical Obstetrics and Gynecology* 43, no. 1 (March 2000): 162–83.

42. Assemi, "Herbs Affecting the Central Nervous System," pp. 824–35.

43. Ibid.

44. Ewies, "A Comprehensive Approach to the Menopause," pp. 642–49.

45. Fredi Kronenberg and Adriane Fugh-Berman, "Complementary and Alternative Medicine for Menopausal Symptoms: A Review of Randomized, Controlled Trials," *Annals of Internal Medicine* 137, no. 10 (November 19, 2002): 805–13.

46. Susan R. Johnson, "Premenstrual Syndrome Therapy," *Clinical Obstetrics and Gynecology* 41, no. 2 (June 1998): 405–21.

47. Kathleen M. Fairfield and Robert H. Fletcher, "Vitamins for Chronic Disease Prevention in Adults: Scientific Review," *Journal of the American Medical Association* 287, no. 23 (June 19, 2002): 3116–26.

48. Ibid.

49. Ibid.

50. Ibid.

51. Katrina M. Wyatt et al., "Efficacy of Vitamin B-6 in the Treatment of Premenstrual Syndrome: Systematic Review," *British Medical Journal* 318, no. 7195 (May 22, 1999): 1375–81.

52. Susan R. Johnson, "Premenstrual Syndrome Therapy," *Clinical Obstetrics and Gynecology* 41, no. 2 (June 1998): 405–21.

53. Fairfield and Fletcher, "Vitamins for Chronic Disease Prevention in Adults," pp. 3116–26.

54. Ibid.

55. Kass-Annese, "Alternative Therapies for Menopause," pp. 162–83.

56. Ligia A. Martini, "Magnesium Supplementation and Bone Turnover," *Nutrition Reviews* 57, no. 7 (July 1999): 227–29.

57. Ibid.

58. F. Facchinetti et al., "Oral Magnesium Successfully Relieves Premen-

strual Mood Changes," *Obstetrics and Gynecology* 78, no. 2 (August 1991): 177–81.

59. F. Facchinetti et al., "Magnesium Prophylaxis of Menstrual Migraine: Effects on Intracellular Magnesium," *Headache* 31, no. 5 (May 1991): 298–301.

60. Gary Nestler and Michael Dovey, "Traditional Chinese Medicine," *Clinical Obstetrics and Gynecology* 44, no. 4 (December 2001): 801–13.

61. Sharon Myoji Schnare, "Complementary and Alternative Medicine: A Primer," *Clinical Obstetrics and Gynecology* 43, no. 1 (March 2000): 157–61.

62. Kronenberg and Fugh-Berman, "Complementary and Alternative Medicine for Menopausal Symptoms," pp. 805–13.

63. Robert S. Mazzeo et al., "ACSM Position Stand: Exercise and Physical Activity for Older Adults," *Medicine and Science in Sports and Exercise* 30, no. 6 (June 1998): 992–1008.

64. Schnare, "Complementary and Alternative Medicine," pp. 157–61.

65. Ibid.

66. Ibid.

67. Ewies, "A Comprehensive Approach to the Menopause," pp. 642–49.

68. J. H. Irvin et al., "The Effects of Relation Response Training on Menopausal Symptoms," *Journal of Psychosomatic Obstetrics and Gynecology* 17, no. 4 (December 1996): 202–207.

69. Ewies, "A Comprehensive Approach to the Menopause," pp. 642–49.

70. Kass-Annese, "Alternative Therapies for Menopause," pp. 162–83.

71. Richard Carter et al., "The Effectiveness of Magnet Therapy for Treatment of Wrist Pain Attributed to Carpal Tunnel Syndrome," *Journal of Family Practice* 51, no. 1 (January 2002): 38–40.

72. Janet S. Carpenter et al., "A Pilot Study of Magnetic Therapy for Hot Flashes after Breast Cancer," *Cancer Nursing* 25, no. 2 (April 2002): 104–109.

CHAPTER 11. LIFE AFTER MENOPAUSE

1. R. R. Recker et al., "Bone Gain in Young Adult Women," *Journal of the American Medical Association* 268 (1992): 2403–2408.

2. L. S. Richelson et al., "Relative Contributions of Aging and Estrogen Deficiency to Postmenopausal Bone Loss," *New England Journal of Medicine* 311 (1984): 1273–75.

3. R. Lindsay, "Prevention and Treatment of Osteoporosis," *Lancet* 341 (1993): 801–805.

4. "Disease Statistics," *National Osteoporosis Foundation* [online], http://www.nof.org/osteoporosis/stats.htm [May 13, 2003].

5. L. J. Melton et al., "How Many Women Have Osteoporosis?" *Journal of Bone and Mineral Research* 7 (1992): 1005–10.

6. S. K. Konar et al., "Factors Associated with Short- vs. Long-Term Skilled Nursing Facility Placement among R. Community-Living Hip Fracture Patients," *Journal of the American Geriatric Society* 38 (1990): 1139–44.

7. P. D. Ross et al., "Pain and Disability Associated with New Vertebral Fractures and Other Spinal Conditions," *Journal of Clinical Epidemiology* 47 (1994): 231–39.

8. Susan Thys-Jacobs et al., "Calcium Carbonate and the Premenstrual Syndrome: Effects on Premenstrual and Menstrual Symptoms," *American Journal of Obstetrics and Gynecology* 179, no. 2 (August 1998): 444–52.

9. Barbara Kass-Annese, "Alternative Therapies for Menopause," *Clinical Obstetrics and Gynecology* 43, no. 1 (March 2000): 162–83.

10. Ligia A. Martini, "Magnesium Supplementation and Bone Turnover," *Nutrition Reviews* 57, no. 7 (July 1999): 227–29.

11. "Osteoporosis: Bone Mass Measurement," *National Osteoporosis Foundation* [online], http://www.nof.org/osteoporosis/bonemass.htm [May 13, 2003].

12. J. A. Griss et al., "Risk Factors for Falls as a Cause of Hip Fracture in Women," *New England Journal of Medicine* 324 (1991): 1326–31.

13. Ayman Ewies, "A Comprehensive Approach to the Menopause: So Far, One Size Should Fit All," *Obstetrical and Gynecological Survey* 56, no. 10 (October 2001): 642–49.

14. B. Lawrence Riggs and Lynn C. Hartmann, "Drug Therapy: Selective Estrogen-Receptor Modulators—Mechanisms of Action and Application to Clinical Practice," *New England Journal of Medicine* 348, no. 7 (February 13, 2003): 618–29.

15. "Facts about Women and Cardiovascular Disease," *American Heart Association* [online], www.americanheart.org [April 3, 2003].

16. Ibid.

17. Lori Mosca et al., "Cardiovascular Disease in Women: A Statement for Healthcare Professionals from the American Heart Association," *Circulation* 96, no. 7 (October 7, 1997): 2468–82.

18. "Heart Attack, Stroke, and Cardiac Arrest Warning Signs," *American Heart Association* [online], www.americanheart.org [April 3, 2003].

19. Pamela Charney, "Presenting Symptoms and Diagnosis of Coronary Heart Disease in Women," *Journal of Cardiovascular Risk* 9, no. 6 (December 2002): 303–307.

20. "Cigarette Smoking–Related Mortality," *Centers for Disease Control and Prevention* [online], www.cdc.gov/tobacco/ [April 7, 2003].

21. "Estimating Coronary Heart Disease (CHD) Risk Using Framingham Heart Study Prediction Score Sheets," *National Heart, Lung, and Blood Institute of the National Institutes of Health* [online], http://www.nhlbi.nih.gov/about/framingham/riskabs.htm [May 8, 2003].

22. Katherine Esposito et al., "Effect of Weight Loss and Lifestyle Changes on Vascular Inflammatory Markers in Obese Women: A Randomized Trial,"

Journal of the American Medical Association 289, no. 14 (April 9, 2003): 1799–1804.

23. Russell R. Pate et al., "Physical Activity and Public Health: A Recommendation from the Centers for Disease Control and Prevention and the American College of Sports Medicine," *Journal of the American Medical Association* 273, no. 5 (February 1, 1995): 402–407; Arne Astrup, "Physical Activity and Weight Gain and Fat Distribution Changes with Menopause: Current Evidence and Research Issues," *Medicine and Science in Sports and Exercise* 31, no. 11 (November 1999): S564.

24. Ibid.

25. Steven N. Blair et al., "Physical Activity, Nutrition, and Chronic Disease," *Medicine and Science in Sports and Exercise* 28, no. 3 (March 1996): 335–49.

26. Robert B. Jaffe, "Physical Activity and Coronary Heart Disease in Women: Is 'No Pain, No Gain' Passé?" *Obstetrical and Gynecological Survey* 56, no. 8 (August 2001): 477–79.

27. Ibid.

28. Frank B. Hu and Walter C. Willett, "Optimal Diets for Prevention of Coronary Heart Disease," *Journal of the American Medical Association* 288, no. 20 (November 27, 2002): 2569–78.

29. Penny M. Kris-Etherton, William S. Harris, and Lawrence J. Appel, "Fish Consumption, Fish Oil, Omega-3 Fatty Acids, and Cardiovascular Disease," *Arteriosclerosis, Thrombosis, and Vascular Biology* 23, no. 2 (February 2003): e20–e30.

30. "An Important Message for Pregnant Women and Women of Childbearing Age Who May Become Pregnant about the Risks of Mercury in Fish," *Revised FDA Consumer Advisory* [online], www.cfsan.fda.gov/seafood1.html [May 7, 2003].

31. Kris-Etherton, Harris, and Appel, "Fish Consumption, Fish Oil, Omega-3 Fatty Acids, and Cardiovascular Disease," pp. e20–e30.

32. Michael J. Thun et al., "Alcohol Consumption and Mortality among Middle-Aged and Elderly U.S. Adults," *New England Journal of Medicine* 337, no. 24 (December 11, 1997): 1705–14.

33. Ian R. White et al., "Alcohol Consumption and Mortality: Modeling Risks for Men and Women at Different Ages," *British Medical Journal* 325, no. 7357 (July 27, 2002): 191–97.

34. J. Rehm et al., "Average Volume of Alcohol Consumption, Patterns of Drinking and Risk of Coronary Heart Disease—A Review," *Journal of Cardiovascular Risk* 10, no. 1 (February 2003): 15–20.

35. White et al., "Alcohol Consumption and Mortality," pp. 191–97.

36. Thun et al., "Alcohol Consumption and Mortality among Middle-Aged and Elderly U.S. Adults," pp. 1705–14; Thomas M. Badger et al., "Alcohol Metabolism: Role in Toxicity and Carcinogenesis," *Alcoholism Clinical and Experimental Research* 27, no. 2 (February 2003): 336–47.

37. Badger et al., "Alcohol Metabolism."

38. Thun et al., "Alcohol Consumption and Mortality among Middle-Aged and Elderly U.S. Adults," pp. 1705–14.

39. Charles Saul Lieber, "Seminars in Medicine of the Beth Israel Hospital, Boston: Medical Disorders of Alcoholism," *Journal of Medicine* 333, no. 16 (October 19, 1995): 1058–65.

40. Robert S. Sandler et al., "A Randomized Trial of Aspirin to Prevent Colorectal Adenomas in Patients with Previous Colorectal Cancer," *New England Journal of Medicine* 348, no. 10 (March 6, 2003): 883–90; Trista W. Johnson et al., "Association of Aspirin and Nonsteroidal Anti-inflammatory Drug Use with Breast Cancer," *Cancer Epidemiology Biomarkers and Prevention* 11 (December 2002): 1586–91; Walter F. Stewart et al., "Risk of Alzheimer's Disease and Duration of NSAID Use," *Neurology* 48, no. 3 (March 1997): 626–32.

41. Michael Hayden et al., "Aspirin for the Primary Prevention of Cardiovascular Events: A Summary of the Evidence for the U.S. Preventive Services Task Force," *Annals of Internal Medicine* 136, no. 2 (January 15, 2002): 161–72.

42. Najib T. Ayas et al., "A Prospective Study of Sleep Duration and Coronary Heart Disease in Women," *Archives of Internal Medicine* 163, no. 2 (January 27, 2003): 205–209.

43. Ibid.

44. "Facts about Women and Cardiovascular Disease," *American Heart Association* [online], www.americanheart.org [April 3, 2003].

45. Harold P. Adams Jr., Gregory J. del Zoppo, and Rudiger von Kummer, *Management of Stroke: A Practical Guide for the Prevention, Evaluation, and Treatment of Acute Stroke* (Caddo, Okla.: Professional Communications, Inc., 1998), p. 32.

CHAPTER 12. SCREENING TESTS

1. "Cancer Facts and Figures 2001," *American Cancer Society* [online], www.cancer.org [May 9, 2003].

2. Ibid.

3. Ibid.

4. Pamela J. Paley, "Ovarian Cancer Screening: Are We Making Any Progress?" *Current Opinion in Oncology* 13, no. 5 (September 2001): 399–402.

5. Ibid.

6. Elizabeth Swisher, M.D., "Hereditary Cancers in Obstetrics and Gynecology," *Clinical Obstetrics and Gynecology* 44 (September 2001): 450–63.

7. Pamela J. Paley, "Screening for the Major Malignancies Affecting Women: Current Guidelines," *American Journal of Obstetrics and Gynecology* 184, no. 5 (April 2001): 1021–30.

8. Ronald T. Burkman et al., "Current Perspectives on Oral Contraceptive Use," *American Journal of Obstetrics and Gynecology* 185, no. 2, supp. (August 2001): S4–S12.

9. "The Role of the Generalist Obstetrician-Gynecologist in the Early Detection of Ovarian Cancer," ACOG Committee Opinion No. 280, *Obstetrics and Gynecology* 100 (December 2002): 1413–16.

10. Ibid.

11. Paley, "Ovarian Cancer Screening: Are We Making Any Progress?" pp. 399–402.

12. Linda L. Humphrey et al., "Breast Cancer Screening: A Summary of the Evidence for the U.S. Preventive Services Task Force," *Annals of Internal Medicine* 135, no. 5 (September 3, 2002): E347–67.

13. Ibid.

14. "Cancer Facts and Figures 2001."

15. Robert S. Sandler et al., "A Randomized Trial of Aspirin to Prevent Colorectal Adenomas in Patients with Previous Colorectal Cancer," *New England Journal of Medicine* 348, no. 10 (March 6, 2003): 883–90.

16. "How Is Colorectal Cancer Found?" *American Cancer Society* [online], www.cancer.org [May 9, 2003].

17. D. A. Lieberman et al., "Use of Colonoscopy to Screen Asymptomatic Adults for Colorectal Cancer. Veterans Affairs Cooperative Study Group," *New England Journal of Medicine* 343 (2000): 162–68.

18. M. Pignone et al., "Screening for Colorectal Cancer in Adults at Average Risk: A Summary of the Evidence for the U.S. Preventive Services Task Force," *Annals of Internal Medicine* 137, no. 2 (July 16, 2002): E132–41.

19. Wendy S. Atkins et al., "Uptake, Yield of Neoplasia, and Adverse Effects of Flexible Sigmoidoscopy," *Gut* 42 (1998): 560–65.

20. R. L. Nelson et al., "Iatrogenic Perforation of the Colon and Rectum," *Diseases of the Colon and Rectum* 25 (1982): 305–308.

21. S. J. Winawer et al., "A Comparison of Colonoscopy and Double-Contrast Barium Enema for Surveillance after Polpectomy," *New England Journal of Medicine* 342 (2000): 393–97.

22. Lieberman et al., "Use of Colonoscopy to Screen Asymptomatic Adults for Colorectal Cancer," pp. 162–68.

23. Pignone et al., "Screening for Colorectal Cancer in Adults at Average Risk," pp. E132–41.

24. Winawer et al., "A Comparison of Colonoscopy and Double-Contrast Barium Enema for Surveillance after Polpectomy," pp. 393–97.

25. "Recommendations and Rationale Screening for Lipid Disorders," *U.S. Preventive Services Task Force* [online], www.ahcpr.gov/clinic/ajpmsuppl/lipidrr.htm [May 9, 2003].

26. "High Blood Cholesterol—What You Need to Know," *National Heart, Lung, and Blood Institute* [online], http://www.nhlbi.nih.gov/health/public/heart/index.htm [May 13, 2003].

27. Ibid.

28. "Recommendations and Rationale Screening for Lipid Disorders."

29. "Live Healthier, Live Longer: Lowering Cholesterol for the Person with Heart Disease," *U.S. Department of Health and Human Services National Cholesterol Education Program* [online], http://www.nhlbi.nih.gov/health/public/heart/chol/liv_chol.htm [May 14, 2003].

30. Ibid.

31. M. J. Bouldin et al., "Quality of Care in Diabetes: Understanding the Guideline," *American Journal of Medical Sciences* 324 (October 2002): 197.

32. Ibid.

33. Erenus Mithat, D. Gurler Aysugul, and Elter Koray, "Should We Consider Performing Oral Glucose Tolerance Tests More Frequently in Postmenopausal Women for Optimal Screening of Impaired Glucose Tolerance?" *Menopause* 9 (July 2002): 297.

34. "American Diabetes Association, Screening for Diabetes: Position Statement," *Diabetes Care* 25 (2002): S21–S24

35. Ibid.

36. Ibid.

37. Swisher, "Hereditary Cancers in Obstetrics and Gynecology," pp. 450–63.

38. Ibid.

39. Ibid.

40. Ibid.

41. Polly A. Marchbanks, et al., "Oral Contraceptives and the Risk of Breast Cancer," *New England Journal of Medicine* 346, no. 26 (June 27, 2002): 2025–32.

42. Swisher, "Hereditary Cancers in Obstetrics and Gynecology," pp. 450–63.

43. Ibid.

44. Ibid.

45. Janet Rose Osuch, M.D., "Breast Health and Disease Over a Lifetime," *Clinical Obstetrics and Gynecology* 45 (December 2002) 1140–61.

46. Swisher, "Hereditary Cancers in Obstetrics and Gynecology," pp. 450–63.

47. Ibid.

48. Ibid.

49. Ibid.

50. Martin Surks, *The Thyroid Book* [online], http://www.thethyroidbook.com/chapter_1.html [May 14, 2003].

51. Paul M. Ridker et al., "Comparison of C-Reactive Protein and Low-Density Lipoprotein Cholesterol Levels in the Prediction of First Cardiovascular Events," *New England Journal of Medicine* 347, no. 20 (November 14, 2002): 1557–65.

52. Michael Hayden et al., "Aspirin for the Primary Prevention of Cardiovascular Events: A Summary of the Evidence for the U.S. Preventive Services Task Force," *Annals of Internal Medicine* 136, no. 2 (January 15, 2002): 161–72.

53. T. S. Church et al., "Associations between Cardiorespiratory Fitness and C-Reactive Protein in Men" *Arteriosclerosis, Thrombosis, and Vascular Biology* 22 (November 2002): 1869–76.

54. Thomas H. Lee and Troyen A. Brennan, "Direct-to Consumer Marketing

of High-Technology Screening Tests," *New England Journal of Medicine* 346 (February 14, 2002): 529–31.

55. Ibid.
56. Ibid.
57. Ibid.

GLOSSARY

adenomyosis. A condition in which part of the lining of the uterus (the endometrium) grows into the uterine walls. Adenomyosis can lead to several problems including painful periods, heavier periods, and pain during intercourse deep in the pelvis.

androgen. The "male" hormones, such as testosterone.

anemia. A deficiency of red blood cells that can be caused by blood loss, a lack of iron, or a deficiency of certain vitamins such as folate or vitamin B12.

Asherman's syndrome. A rare condition in which the inner walls of the uterus scar together.

Body Mass Index (BMI). A measurement that uses height and weight to calculate a number that provides a more accurate measure of total body fat than using weight alone.

CA-125. A blood test that is sometimes used to detect ovarian cancer.

colposcopy. A procedure in which the vaginal walls and cervix are examined with a colposcope after an abnormal Pap smear. The colposcope is basically a microscope that gives a close-up view of the cervix so that any abnormalities can be better seen. Biopsies may be done at the same time as the colposcopy to determine more precisely the nature of the abnormal Pap smear.

deep vein thrombosis (DVT). A blood clot in the deep veins of the legs.

dilation and curettage (D&C). A surgical procedure in which the cervix is dilated and the lining of the uterus is scraped.

dysfunctional uterine bleeding. Abnormal bleeding from the uterus that is not caused by a physical or medical problem. This diagnosis is made only after the woman has been evaluated and after other causes for bleeding have been eliminated.

emboli. A plug or mass such as a blood clot or air bubble that travels through the bloodstream and becomes lodged, thus blocking a blood vessel.

endometrial ablation. A procedure in which the lining of the uterus is destroyed to help decrease menstrual bleeding.

endometrial biopsy. A procedure usually done in the physician's office in which a narrow tube is placed in the uterus, suction is applied, and a sample of the lining of the uterus is obtained.

endometrial hyperplasia. A condition in which there is an overgrowth of the lining of the uterus.

endometrial polyp. A growth, usually benign, that arises from the endometrial (uterine) lining.

endometriosis. A condition in which the endometrium, the lining of the uterus, grows outside of the uterus—where it's not supposed to be. Endometriosis may cause inflammation and pain.

estrogen. A "female" hormone that is produced mainly by the ovaries. Estrogen is responsible for developing the female reproductive system, for the changes seen during puberty, and for stimulating the lining of the uterus during the menstrual cycle.

fibroid. Also called leiomyoma, is a common benign growth in the uterus. It arises from the smooth muscle cells in the wall of the uterus and can grow anywhere in the uterus, from the inside lining, to deep in the wall, or on the outer surface.

fistula. An abnormal opening between two organs or an organ and the skin. For example an opening between the bowel and vagina causing stool to leak through the vagina.

Follicle Stimulating Hormone (FSH). Hormone produced by the pituitary gland, a small gland at the base of the brain. It stimulates the ovaries to produce estrogen.

Gonadotropin Releasing Hormone (GnRH agonist). Medication that is used to shut down the ovaries, causing a temporary state of menopause.

hematocrit. A blood test for anemia that measures the percentage of red blood cells in the blood.

hormone. A chemical made in one part of the body that affects cells in other areas of the body. Hormones act as messengers, carrying information and instructions that may have local or general effects.

hyperthyroidism. A condition in which the thyroid produces too much thyroid hormone.

hypothyroidism. A condition in which the thyroid produces too little thyroid hormone.

hysterectomy. A surgical procedure in which the uterus is removed.

hysteroscopy. A procedure where a hysteroscope, a telescope-type instrument, is used to look inside the uterus.

laparoscopy. A procedure where a laparoscope, a telescope-type instrument, is used to look inside the pelvis and abdomen.

menopause. The time when a woman stops menstruating because of a loss of functioning of her ovaries. The average age of menopause in this country is fifty-one, with most women going through menopause between the ages of forty-eight and fifty-five.

myomectomy. A procedure where fibroids are removed from the uterus.

nonsteroidal anti-inflammatory drug (NSAID). An anti-inflammatory medication such as ibuprofen, aspirin, and naproxen.

osteoporosis. A progressive disease in which the bones get so thin and weak that they can break easily.

Pap smear. A screening test for cervical cancer done by collecting cervical cells with a spatula and a brush. The cells are sent to a lab where they are analyzed.

perimenopause. The time leading up to menopause when women start to have symptoms related to this time of transition.

postmenopause. The time after the last menstrual period. Postmenopause lasts for the rest of a woman's life.

premature menopause. This term refers to women going through menopause early. Some people define premature menopause as menopause before age thirty-five, while others say before age forty. About 1 percent of women go through menopause under the age of forty. This is due to the ovaries in these women failing prematurely.

premenstrual dysphoric disorder (PMDD). A severe form of PMS that meets certain criteria.

premenstrual syndrome (PMS). Bothersome symptoms that affect a woman one to two weeks before the onset of her period.

progesterone. A "female" hormone that is produced mainly by the ovaries with a small amount made by the adrenal gland.

progestin. A synthetic compound that acts like progesterone.

Selective Estrogen-Receptor Modulator (SERM). Medication that acts like estrogen in one area of the body and like an antiestrogen in other parts of the body. Tamoxifen and raloxifene are the two examples of SERMs.

serotonin reuptake inhibitors (SSRIs). A class of antidepressants that are thought to work by improving serotonin activity in the brain. Drugs in this class include fluoxetine (Prozac), paroxetine (Paxil), sertraline (Zoloft), citalopram (Celexa), and venlafaxine (Effexor).

sonohysterogram (Saline Infusion Sonography). A procedure in which a small, flexible plastic tube called a catheter is placed inside the uterus. Fluid is placed through the catheter into the uterus enabling the ultrasound to detect any abnormal growths inside the uterus such as polyps and fibroids.

testosterone. A "male" hormone. In a woman, testosterone promotes sex drive, builds up bones and muscles, and helps with feelings of general well-being.

thrombophlebitis. Inflammation of a vein caused by a blood clot.

uterine artery embolization. A procedure whereby the major arteries to the uterus are blocked. It is usually done to cause large fibroids to shrink.

vaginismus. A condition in which the muscles around the opening to the vagina become so tight that intercourse becomes painful.

INDEX